FREUD AND THE CHANGING WORLD

FREUD AND
THE CHANGING WORLD

Contemporary Psychoanalysis
and Its Troubles

Stefano Bolognini and Luca Nicoli

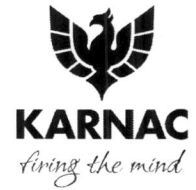

KARNAC
firing the mind

Originally published in 2022 in Italian as *Freud e il mondo che cambia. Psicoanalisi del presente e dei suoi guai* by Enrico Damiani Editore e Associati

First published in English in 2025 by
Karnac Books Limited
62 Bucknell Road
Bicester
Oxfordshire OX26 2DS

British Library Cataloguing in Publication Data

A C.I.P. for this book is available from the British Library

ISBN: 978-1-80013-280-1 (paperback)
ISBN: 978-1-80013-279-5 (e-book)
ISBN: 978-1-80013-278-8 (PDF)

Typeset by vPrompt eServices Pvt Ltd, India

Printed in the United Kingdom

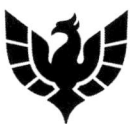

www.firingthemind.com

Contents

Acknowledgements

The conversation at the centre of Chapter 4, "Soul and body", was prompted by and refers to two books that I consider illuminating of Stefano Bolognini's thought, *Vital Flows Between the Self and Non-Self: The Interpsychic* (Routledge, 2022) and *Secret Passages: The Theory and Technique of Interpsychic Relations* (Routledge, 2011): a collection of texts of extraordinary clinical and theoretical interest as well as of rare practical utility.

Chapter 9, "Offline and online", takes its cue from "What we have learned: A conversation with Stefano Bolognini"—Report by Pietro Roberto Goisis and Silvio A. Merciai from *Covid-19 Pandemic and Online Therapy* published in 2021 in *Gamma Function* (48), https://www.funzionegamma.it/en/covid-19-pandemic-and-online-therapy/.

About the authors

Stefano Bolognini is a psychiatrist and a training and supervising analyst of the Italian Psychoanalytic Society (SPI). He is the former President of the SPI and past President of the International Psychoanalytical Association (IPA), after having been IPA board representative for two mandates and member and chair of several IPA committees. He is a former member of the European editorial board of the *International Journal of Psychoanalysis* and of the European Psychoanalytical Federation (EPF) theoretical working party. He is also an honorary member of the New York Contemporary Freudian Society (CFS), the Los Angeles Institute and Society for Psychoanalytic Studies (LAISPS), and the Florence Psychoanalytic Center (CPF), and a member of the advisory board of the International Psychoanalytic University of Berlin (IPU). He was the founder of the IPA *Inter-Regional Encyclopedic Dictionary of Psychoanalysis* (IRED) and former chair. He has published over 280 psychoanalytic papers and eight books, including *Vital Flows Between the Self and Non-Self: The Interpsychic* (Routledge, 2022), which won the 2023 Gradiva Award. Dr Bolognini lives and works in Bologna, Italy.

Luca Nicoli is a full member of the Italian Psychoanalytic Society (SPI) and the International Psychoanalytical Association (IPA). He was formerly an Adjunct Professor at the Faculty of Psychology, University of Parma, and is currently a lecturer at the AION Specialisation School of Psychodynamic Therapy in Bologna. He has been an editorial member of the *Italian Journal of Psychoanalysis*, and is currently a reviewer for the *International Journal of Psychoanalysis*. He has published in Italian and international scientific journals, as well as several psychoanalytic books. The popular book *The New Analyst's Guide to the Galaxy: Questions about Contemporary Psychoanalysis*, co-written with Antonino Ferro (Karnac, 2017), has been translated into five languages.

Preface

Paul Newman, patient 2.0, and our present

I t is with great pleasure that I introduce the reader to the discovery of this book, a text capable of meeting both the attention of the professional audience and the curiosity of anyone who wants to take a look, even for the first time, at the world of psychoanalysis. The questioning acumen of Luca Nicoli, a pioneer in the field of a new genre of nonfiction, that of "Interviews with the Masters of Contemporary Psychoanalysis", solicits Stefano Bolognini's thought, his clinical and institutional experience, and his psychoanalytic wisdom into dialogue. Out of this encounter comes a work of lively discussion, captivating and enthralling the reader in the exploration of crucial and highly topical issues.

Bolognini, with his trademark grace, clarity, depth, and strictness, takes us on a close observation of psychoanalysis. He highlights the changes in clinical practice and theory that have happened over the past century, since Sigmund Freud devised a method of knowledge and treatment capable of going beyond the appearances of human behaviour, initiating an epistemological revolution in the understanding of the individual's psychiatric functioning and its psychopathological drifts, personality development, and relational life. At the centre, and at the foundation of everything, is the recognition of the existence of the dynamic unconscious, a dimension of the psyche inescapable for any reflection on psychoanalysis.

In the dialogue between Bolognini and Nicoli, the attention to the constituent nucleus of the analytic experience is always central: the development, in the therapeutic relationship, of a particular intimacy, functional to the cure, between a human being who becomes a "patient", with his suffering and his request for help, and another human being, the analyst, endowed with a professional competence conjugated to his most authentic personal presence. Two people who talk in a room, "an encounter between two persons" as captured by Luciana Nissim Momigliano: two people who, for several years, meet regularly defining a very special relationship, through which the patient has the possibility of finding a way out of the blind alleys of anguish, improving his mental functioning and the quality of relationship with himself and others.

To better illustrate the meaning of these considerations, I bring back a clinical episode with a patient of mine who was nearing the end of treatment. After several years of sessions, which began with pervasive anguish over great difficulty in relationships with women, he told me about a dream in which he sees himself in the mirror with the face of Paul Newman. In all evidence, although he was a man of pleasant appearance, his aesthetics were decidedly far from the loveliness of the famous Hollywood actor, but there was no need for any particular interpretative contortions in search of grandiose fantasies of beauty, seductive capacities towards the female sex, or envious attacks on an idealised and unattainable oedipal rival. The dream interpreted itself, so to speak, and spoke explicitly to us of its new condition, of the changes that had become entrenched in the inner world of that patient, who happened to be named Paul …

The red thread of a reflection on contemporaneity is what guides the development of all the chapters of this book: both in referring to the characteristics and critical issues that define the global context in which we live, and in pointing out clearly what it can mean to "do psychoanalysis" today. The authors give us back a picture of psychoanalysis in step with the times, contradicted by theoretical and technical innovations that allow clinical practice to be declined in the context of a human reality, individual and social, profoundly different from that of its origins.

The reader can easily understand what it means, today, to be a patient and what being an analyst entails.

I will point out, for the less experienced, that the psychoanalyst is entitled to the competence of a working method acquired during a long training, theoretical and clinical, of study and experience, which leads him or her to undergo first-hand a long and careful analysis, without which he or she is not qualified to apply the same process to his or her patients.

Bolognini and Nicoli tell us that psychoanalysis is far from being in crisis, or even dead, as a certain and recurring (sub)cultural tendency with a scientistic imprint would have us believe. On the contrary, psychoanalysis still has much to offer, and its challenge is to intercept new needs and new forms of suffering, and to propose modes of intervention that contemporary subjectivities can follow.

An example is provided by the references in the book to the complexity of the work the analyst has to do in defining the analytic setting and in ensuring its resilience, including the discourse of online analysis, which, unsurprisingly, the global Covid-19 pandemic led us to experience. The setting, for today's analyst, cannot give itself exclusively as a framework pre-constituted from established technocratic prescriptions, but must be carefully constructed, respecting on the one hand the singularities of the patient, and on the other hand the needs for invariance inherent in the psychoanalytic method. It is increasingly essential to be able to make adjustments to the setting that try to ensure the best possible analytic work for each specific clinical experience. The viability of an analysis is to be defined by the contributions of the patient, who tends to "stay in the setting" according to the determinants of his or her mental structure and specific relational modes. And, on this point, "patient 2.0" imposes new stresses that necessitate inevitable readjustments of the analyst's theoretical and co-technical toolkit.

In this sense, this book does not renege on the promise of its title, *Freud and the Changing World*. The contents get straight to the point, offering a psychoanalytic look at contemporaneity and the difficulties that afflict individuals' emotional lives and the quality of interpersonal relationships today. We find here many of the themes dear to Stefano Bolognini: empathy, analytic intimacy, the interpsychic, the dialectic between the centred ego and the experiential self (in the patient and the analyst), the importance of the preconscious, the different types of transference, relational action, new modes of interpretation, to name but a few. As a testimony to the widespread interest in psychoanalysis, I would add that *Freud and the Changing World* is also the name of a successful popularisation initiative that, for over ten years, together with Luca Nicoli, we have been carrying out in the territory of the province of Modena, with the lively participation of a very heterogeneous public.

One aspect that guarantees particular enjoyment in reading this book is the skilful use of metaphors and references to everyday situations that, in their easy and immediate usability, effectively represent the complexities of psychic functioning and relational interactions. Bolognini, in recounting significant episodes of personal experience, shows us how it is possible, as well as desirable, to achieve that process of integration which lies at the base of a healthy professional identity: the integration between one's own human subjectivity and the theoretical–clinical options, profoundly and authentically assimilated, as the foundation of the possibility of exercising a valid analytic function finalised to patient care.

One final note. In the argumentative developments of the book, the dialogue between Bolognini and Nicoli generates a discursive plot charged with an emotional intensity that shows us a "thinking and feeling together" which constitutes, among other things, the qualifying datum of the very experience that takes place between patient and analyst. A captivating dialogue and a fertile confrontation between two different generations of analysts is eloquent testimony to how psychoanalysis can keep pace with our present and, through transformation and evolution in theory and clinical practice, can take us into the future.

My thanks, therefore, to Stefano Bolognini and Luca Nicoli. And, to you, good reading!

Stefano Tugnoli
Medical psychiatrist, SPI psychoanalyst, and Adjunct Professor
at the University of Ferrara

A note from the authors

Dear reader

In reporting our conversation on the written page, we have used our initials, SB for Stefano Bolognini and LN for Luca Nicoli, to show who is speaking. At all times, we try to use accessible language, limiting the use of technical/scientific terms to only where it is essential.

Where it proves necessary to use more technical terms, wherever possible, we clarify the terminology in the text. Where terms require further explanation, we refer the reader to a glossary at the back of the book.

Words and expressions explained in the glossary are indicated by an asterisk (*) the first time they appear in the text.

We hope that this system facilitates the flow of the text to make an enjoyable reading experience, whilst, at the same time, giving a helping hand to those approaching psychoanalytic theory for the first time.

Stefano Bolognini and Luca Nicoli

CHAPTER 1

The troubles of the present

LN: Psychoanalysis has turned 120 years old. In some ways it has changed a lot, in others it retains close connections with its origins. In your opinion, what is the most precious legacy it carries with it, which you couldn't do without?

SB: I think that the exploration of the unconscious, although today it is done "with" the patient whilst in the past it was more "about" the patient, has remained in spirit consistent with the origins of psychoanalysis. The setting*—which we continue, as far as possible under normal circumstances, to keep well-structured and rhythmically constant— is also an element of continuity, because it helps to work in precisely this direction. There are a great many other aspects that characterise the legacy we received from the founders, but this device is substantial (and for that matter, precisely because of its scenic power, it has been scoped far and wide by the imitators of psychoanalysis).

The ways in which such exploration takes place today, instead, are perhaps a little different from their origins. Freud asked his patients to cooperate, confiding in the analyst their free associations,* as we do too, because we place a great deal of importance on what the patient says, what comes into his mind, how he tells us, and so on.

For a long time, however, the analyst saw himself or herself as a mirror, who had to do and say as little as possible, whereas today we take it for granted that the process is more complex and that the analyst, however reserved and abstinent, also does something, whether he or she wants to or not.

The analyst does something with his or her way of waiting, of being completely silent or intervening, of providing the patient with his or her associations or keeping them to himself or herself. He does something in creating the "aspirational" vacuum—of waiting and listening sensitively and willingly, or by making one's own withdrawal felt—which are two quite different things—and so on.

So, there are many points of continuity with the early technique, but there are also important novelties and variations.

However, the analytic process, with its developments, has remained a vantage point: with a part of our mind at work, we resonate "short-range" to the patient's words by associating in turn; in parallel, however, we maintain a focus on the process unfolding in the medium and long term, and observe what happens over time, over sessions, months, years.

A great deal of attention has been paid to the effects of the absences of the object* (in our case of the analyst), to their consequences on the more primitive parts of the patient, which are common to all patients, including the more evolved and more acculturated ones: it could be said that as human beings we are all similar—though not the same—when faced with the vicissitudes of the presence or absence of an object.

Of course, some react more acutely or with greater suffering, others apparently do not, but the oscillations in the object relationship—how we relate to the other in the face of the fundamental factor of its presence or absence—we all experience them; it varies greatly, however, the degree of individual awareness regarding this experience.

In my opinion, an important element that has changed in this century is our increased awareness of normal human physiology in the psychic field.

Whereas once psychoanalysis was strongly attracted to psychic pathology and dealt primarily with that, to solve its impenetrable mystery today we know, with greater "democratic" resignation, that there is a basic physiology common to all human beings, in all their object relations. Analysts, too, experience relational fluctuations in their relationships, approaches and withdrawals, neither more nor less with others. On the contrary, precisely because of having gotten in touch earlier, through their personal analysis, with their own otherwise unconscious psychological vicissitudes, they can help others become more familiar with these internal developments and movements that are not easy for an inexperienced subject to read.

The analyst, after all, is a person who knows these passages a little more than his or her patient and, if things have gone well enough, has become familiar with these ways of living and being.

It used to be that the analyst's gaze was more entomological, that is, he looked at the patient a bit from above, recognising his anomalies with more detachment.

LN: You mentioned the absence of the object as one of the main problems to be addressed for the psychic growth of the individual. Can you tell us about that?

SB: It is. The absence of the object is the testing ground of the subject's* capacity to wait for its return, maintaining or not maintaining an internal, affective, and representational* bond with it: for example, retaining the ability to think about a person who is not there, instead of closing that drawer and acting as if it doesn't exist until it returns (and sometimes even afterwards ...).

In other cases, the absent object is immediately replaced with another, so as not to feel the pain of absence. There is a huge range of defensive solutions in the face of the absence of the object, which makes it easier not to think about it. In the American films of the 1960s, much was played of the joke of the wife on vacation or the husband in town.

One saw husbands who somewhat maniacally set out on the hunt for alternative objects, more or less like Sylvester the cat who sets out to catch the house canary as soon as the mistress is absent: with zero awareness, in many cases, of the fact that the increase in the number of revolutions of the internal motor, i.e. the hypomanic regime*, was an unconscious defensive reaction to not feel and not suffer the absence of the object.

Mind you, in some cases, there is also a genuine search for a sense of freedom in such extramarital adventures, for example, when the spouse is too oppressive, too inhibiting; but a good portion of these reckless escapades have this defensive function.

LN: In other words, these summer hunts had and have the unconscious objective of covering up the pain of lack, replacing it with manic excitement…

SB: Yes. We in analysis detect these defensive processes enacted against us quite frequently. In fact, it often happens that during the first summer separation the patients, still well-defended, do not feel so much the lack of the analysis and the analyst, whilst from the second summer break they begin to feel the weight of the absence; and the longer it goes on, year after year, the more they feel it. In a sense, the separation of the first year is often little felt because the patient has little internal contact with their own deep experiences: which explains the apparent paradox of their being less anguished at the detachment.

Of course, it is also true that over time patients learn to bear it better without losing the relationship, without losing the internal bond, being able to trust that we will meet again: when things work sufficiently well, this is how it is.

In the beginning, on the other hand, patients' resistance* to experiencing sorrow and grief when missing the object is very high; besides the fact that they often do not attribute depression over the long summer separation to the absence of analysis, but to the most diverse of causes.

In ordinary life, outside the analytic context, the same thing can happen, that is, that the bond, the affective bond with an object, is almost forgotten and locked in a drawer so as not to feel bad when the object is not there; this can be done in a hypomanic way with so many diversionary manoeuvres, from the clandestine summer "hunts" I mentioned earlier, to substance use, to paroxysmal abuse of technology.

After all, putting up with the thought that the object is not there, thinking about it, remembering it, is not an obvious attitude, in today's way of life.

It used to be that people wrote to each other by mail, knowing that the letter would arrive to the beloved or loved one only after a few days; one had to prepare for the wait. Now with mobile phones this is no longer the case; everything is instantaneous. Moreover, today's society gives us many opportunities to create anti-objects or alternative objects to the basic one that replaces it when it is missing, thus circumventing the suffering from absence; thus we get those situations that I call "of the catamaran or trimaran" (the sail boats with two or three hulls), in which one puts one foot here and one foot over there, distributing and balancing between several relationships at once in order not to suffer.

LN: We could say that the avoidance of pain is the backbone of this society of ours.

SB: I think so. Once upon a time, a good support for enduring loneliness was provided by religion, because it suggested the idea that someone "up there" (God, Our Lady, saints, equivalents of adult parental figures; or the Guardian Angel, another self) was always there and always thinking of us, and that we could contact him or her in a private, other, highly invested emotional reality on the plane of faith. Today as religion is generally much less invested in, other concrete ways for object substitution are sought.

LN: Pain avoidance, object substitutions during its absence, manic reactions to depressive feelings, even non-pathological ones. With such an average psychic setup, it is no surprise that psychic suffering is kept at a distance from consciousness, without experiencing and acknowledging it. The stigma of mental illness is still found in common thinking. There are many myths to dispel: there is the idea of the insane person as someone who is broken. They used to be called alienated, to emphasise that they were out of their minds. Then there's the idea of willpower, which is mostly about depression: "That guy can't get out of it on his own because he doesn't want to, he doesn't try hard enough to succeed". Plus there's a whole issue of children. Children are mostly diagnosed according to the criteria of "specific learning disorders", as if to reiterate an exclusive interest in the efficiency of the child-pupil. Or they are hyperactive, and the focus is on their behaviour rather than on their interiority. Adolescents, on the other hand, are not infrequently regarded as lazy or rude, whilst states of depressive anguish, physiological at this age, sometimes accentuated by deeper turmoil and anguish, are still unrecognised.

This whole roundup of stereotypical views shows how much prejudice still hovers around mental suffering. In your opinion, how can we define mental illness?

SB: Mental illness unfortunately exists; it is an outcome that is real, although there are still those who would ideologically tend to deny it, blaming suffering only on social difficulties, lack of willpower, and so on. What is often missing—and what analysts can help recreate—is, on the cultural and even the scientific level, an understandable continuity, a bridge between physiology and pathology.

When dealing with a very pathologic person, the tendency of most laymen is either to deny the pathology altogether by laughing about it, or commenting that "That's just the way he is", "He's a weirdo", "He's an original" (phrases that were once heard, especially in the countryside); or—bouncing to the opposite extreme—that of thinking that the person is hopelessly insane and says things that make no sense at all.

It is true that there are borderline psychopathological conditions with such a level of psychic destruction that it becomes very difficult to identify the broken bridge between pathology and physiology, to reconstruct how one could have arrived at such an altered internal world*, and to attempt to initiate some partial process of repair, or at least of management and adaptation. However, it is also true that, in principle, analysts have more experience, honed through work on themselves, of the transitions between the physiological and the pathological. Put another way: psychoanalysts are better able than others to figure out how a sufficiently healthy and integrated person can decompensate, in certain situations, to the point of appearing completely altered and lacking a contact with reality.

Here it is: analysts of that path between physiology and pathology (both outward and, sometimes, thank goodness, backwards), know it a little better because of their subjective experience of regression*, experienced in their analysis.

Even, it seems that in the 1950s and early 1960s, the joke ran among analysts that one should not select as future students people who were too healthy, because they would become therapists who were incapable of negotiating the road, the path, the underground workings between being healthy and being sick.

Those who had gone through a very disturbing experience and had managed to emerge from it, thanks to analytic treatment with better knowledge of the path of possible restoration: they were like a mountain guide who had already experienced in their own skin many of the passages that their clients/patients would have to face.

To me, this sounds like a nice metaphor, because it gives the idea of how analytic competence is based not only on theories, which are also useful and serve as a guide, but also on lived experiences on one's own, with one's Self*.

LN: Your answer clarifies what an analyst is and how he or she differs from other mental health workers. You did not give me an answer as a psychiatrist, which you are, nor an answer as a diagnostician. You did not speak of categories, of criteria and malfunctions, all of which you know very well, of how damaged or suffering the self or the psychic container* can be.

Rather, your emphasis on the continuity between human functioning gives us the image of analyst and patient understood as two people who are in the same boat and share the same difficulties: neither is an alien nor a stowaway to be repatriated. There is a lost sense to be recovered through collaboration and sharing states that are too difficult to live alone.

SB: Yes, the famous Terentian phrase "*Homo sum, nihil humani mihi alienum puto*" ("I am a human and therefore I consider nothing human alien to me") can be evoked even in the face of very altered conditions of the psyche.

Not that in order to be an analyst one has to complete the training with a forced hospitalisation to experience what psychotic unrest is; however, it is certain that all of us, if we are sincere enough to admit it, have experienced from within the functional fluctuations of the ego*, the occasional detachment from ourselves, despair, fury.

The analyst knows the "regressive pits", those phases or moments when the functional tone drops, the confidence in oneself crumbles, and dependence on the other becomes total and painful, combined with a sense of helplessness; the analyst can also recognise in others and in oneself the projective and paranoid overtones from which no one is absolutely exempt. There is not a person in the world to whom this has not happened.

The Kleinian school* described these projective and paranoid overtones better than others, recognising these defence mechanisms* as something universal, obviously with very important differences in quantity and effects.

Now, as you and I converse, we are about to resume work after the summer, and we know very well how this will implicate, in the first weeks of sessions, the gathering of the resonances* and consequences of the summer absence of the object: an experience of separation that will procure, as we have mentioned, at first a sense of emotional distancing in many patients, who will come back to the session seemingly without any particular reaction. But this is only appearance. In later sessions, all the turbulence resulting from the experience of lack will come out, and we will find this tension in them both in their relationship with us and in their relationship with significant external figures. And after that again we will come, if all goes well, to contact with the healthy pain, the one endowed with meaning and consciously connected to the experience of the lack of the object, of the other; and then we can begin to reinforce and heal the separative fracture, heal the wound of detachment, and so on.

These are universal processes that used to be less known about.

Of course, Freud spoke of the "Monday scab", referring to the tighter defences he found in patients after the weekend break; today, after a century of psychoanalytic practice, we are better equipped and more familiar with these fluctuations, which spare no one.

LN: Doctor, the taboo of the early years of the last century was sexuality. What do you think is the taboo of today?

SB: I think it is the internal dialectics of individuals with their Ego Ideal, the psychic instance that tells us how we would like and/or should be. The biggest fear is not being okay, not living up to it, not being lovable, admirable, maybe even enviable.

Today, the ideal role model may be a beautiful actor or actress, a highly successful figure, the trumpeter, the billionaire sportsman, the influencer, and so on: these are figures with a high rate of aestheticisation and narcissistic* enhancement. For goodness sake, they are also bearers of qualities that have their own value; mind you, they should not be denigrated in a moralistic manner; however, they are in danger of becoming structuring clichés and of imposing ironclad parameters of evaluation.

A patient told me that there are token websites in which grades are given according to defined and targeted criteria that end up giving a specific score to each person. They put together several criteria, not just one.

It seems that the scores of these sites are very approximate, sort of like when kids used to test their strength at the amusement park by punching a mechanical punchbag that measured their ability. Today these sites dispense a quantitative value, an overall score to the qualities, characteristics, and achievements of people in various areas: beauty, wealth, social ability, and so on. This creates a ruthless comparative reality, in which the Ideal Ego inevitably becomes persecutory.

Such an operation was accomplished *de facto* so many years ago with the measurement of IQ: some international associations allowed access to their club only to people who scored above a certain mark. However, today, it seems to me, there is a further stage of dangerous dehumanisation, and we are still there: guilt has been replaced by shame, the experiences of inferiority, unworthiness, and inadequacy. The moral character of the superego*, once the natural enemy of psychoanalysts, is now less strong; instead, the Ego Ideal has become overwhelming and pervasive, the real master of the stage.

LN: One would say that times change, treatments are refined, but diseases remain the same. Gastric ulcers, high blood pressure, influenza do not change over the centuries. Living conditions are different today; in so much of the world, fortunately, the diseases of malnutrition no longer exist or they are disappearing: pellagra, the scurvy that afflicted the sailors of Columbus and Magellan. Other diseases have been eradicated thanks to vaccines, or cures, or surgery, with others that we now live with for longer than in the past; they become chronic. We can see cases of this right before our eyes in the present. Have mental illnesses changed?

SB: Observing changes in psychopathologies through the decades is not a new exercise; Eugenio Gaddini's (1984) observations in the 1980s have remained classic, when he noted a number of changes, in fact already clearly visible then, compared to previous decades.

As we have said, in the first part of the century the great defendant in psychoanalysis was often, if not always, the superego, insofar as it prevented the ego from a serene dialectic with drives*, memories, fantasies, and in general with the repressed*. Remorse that, instead of being acknowledged and more or less dealt with consciously, was censored and repressed: certain things should not even be thought of. Many of the most prevalent neurotic forms were the result of the dominance of a too-strong censor apparatus, which prevented the subject from knowing and dealing with his own internal conflicts.

Psychoanalysis shone a conscious beam of light on the deep-seated polemics and inner struggles of its patients, responsibly confronting them with the internal tensions by which they were not only torn apart (which is part of the normal human condition), but which the patients themselves tried to evade, not to acknowledge.

Undoubtedly there has been, with time, a conspicuous decline in the frequency of certain forms of neurosis*, for example, the major obsessive neuroses. Even very widespread phobias have declined, gradually transforming into new forms: for example, the area of "limit pathology", that is, the difficulty of recognising limits and accepting them, has expanded greatly. It used to be that many patients had to be helped to overcome their inhibitions: the drive-machine only released a weak amount of horsepower to run the engine, or more often the engine was restrained by a constantly engaged inhibitory handbrake; today, conversely, there is a certain insufficiency in the braking system.

Then there is the whole question concerning identity complexity, for example, regarding gender identity, the high degree of articulation of which is now recognised—with greater finesse and less prejudice. The risk on the horizon may be, if anything, that of an excess of fascination towards a kind of virtual omnipotence, whereby one pretends not to have an identity profile of any kind, instead of coming to terms with a profile that is perhaps very complex and very unusual, but which, however, corresponds well or badly to the actual reality of the subject.

It seems, however, that preserving a sense of omnipotence is becoming a general aspiration; which does not mean recognising new, different, or less compliant identities from the past that demand to exist as they feel and are. No, there is something more. There is a claim to a "non-definiteness" of nothing, a being able to change oneself continuously and at will, a deliberately wanting to be protean, even with a certain complacency. This is always part of the pathology of the limit, in which one thinks that limits should not be there and that they may not exist; which is unrealistic on the plane of real life.

LN: In this regard, you pointed out certain social changes that may have contributed to the evolution of a narcissistic sense of people's relational style.

SB: In my opinion, one of the elements—within a complex multifactoriality that is changing our lives—is the primary relationship with the object experienced today by newborns and infants: changes within this relationship have been risking for several years that the relational centre of gravity of the baby is instinctively withdrawing from the investigation of the mother to the one towards the self. I do not exclude that this is precisely one of the great psychosocial elements that have changed in the last forty to fifty years.

I have identified two macro-factors with regard to this scope, and here I know that I am going to touch on delicate situations: one is that most mothers today are working, which is fine from a thousand points of view. The crucial step, however, is the length of time spent with the child before going back to work, because contractually many of them have to go back too early, and the symbiotic, physiological function with the little one is broken very early.

The infant in the beginning is totally dependent on maternal care and on intense, fusional psychic and bodily contact, which allows it to maintain for a time some continuity with the intrauterine foetal condition. This high level of fusionality naturally decreases as the weeks and months go by; it is what I like to call a "soft landing", a process that must be gradual to succeed best. If the initial physiological fusionality is interrupted too soon or too abruptly, this can disrupt the integration of the forming subject: and the first effect may be that of a partial defensive withdrawal of affective investment in the mother-object, with a narcissistic retreat of the infant back onto itself.

I am aware that this is a politically incorrect thesis. There is no absolute standard that establishes on a scientific basis, and in a precise way, how long a mother should be with the child before returning to work, all the more so when one considers not only the "how much" but especially the "how" of the initial fusional cohabitation experience.

Some customs in our Western world, according to which mothers return to the office full-time a month or two after giving birth, however, are at odds with the physiological fusional needs of newborns; and so is the fact that there is not, in many cases, a fairly stable and constant integrative figure to support the children. Childcare provision is a revolving door: carers disappear as they appear, for a thousand reasons that are more than understandable from a socio-economic point of view, but with traumatic discontinuity for the little ones.

The second factor is the macro-phenomenon of nuclear families, which no longer have the outline and support of those of origin. The figures of family members (grandparents, uncles, cousins), which used to be stable elements in large peasant homes (let us not forget that until the late 1950s, 70 per cent of Italian families lived from agriculture) and which created a stable growing environment for the child, are no longer there today.

Married couples have gained a great deal in terms of freedom, so perhaps the overall balance is good in the end. We all know how much phantasmatic intrigue, how many bloody conflicts, and how many subterranean tensions were created, for example, between mothers-in-law and daughters-in-law, or between brothers-in-law: real relational hells curbed in their explosive potential by the dictates of upbringing or religion, but which today would not be contained, nor tolerated in the same way.

On the other hand, those who have gained the least—indeed, frankly lost—from this reduction of parental networks are the children, in case they cannot count on substitute caregivers—stable caregivers, like, for example, grandparents. And this is no small problem.

When grandparents are constant figures in a child's life, the fact that the mother is not so much at home is compensated for rather well; if there is a rotation of caregivers, on the other hand, the subject instinctively (and not because he or she is lucidly reasoning about it, which he or she is often not even capable of doing) retreats in on himself or herself. It's as if the subject (the child) is saying to the object, "I know you're going to leave anyway, I know you're going to change and someone else is going to come; and so I'm going to do things on my own".

Dear Dr Nicoli, think of the association I get when re-looking at the constancy of the object … Once upon a time, football teams had flag players. Rivera for Milan, Di Stefano for Real Madrid, Cruyff for Ajax. In every city in Europe, in the big teams, a charismatic symbol-figure stood out who was the pivot of affective and identity reference for the fans. Today there is such a whirlwind of football players that the fan has a hard time picturing his or her team in a clearly defined way: the flag-bearers are almost gone; today, football players spin like spinning tops from one team to another in pursuit of the most lucrative signings.

Babysitters tend to behave in the same way, converting themselves into globetrotters of the primary relationship; only that whilst the loss of flag-bearers does not produce serious consequences, even if the mass of supporters is the equivalent of a regressed subject, for a child in the primary stage to see a babysitter-object change every few months is not the same thing.

LN: Is this not the same thing that is also noticed by analysts when they meet the children they have treated when they have grown up.

SB: When they go to the analyst—and here we come to us—Millennials are told that they would need intensive, continuous, long-term treatment, which concretely means: "Dear patient, if you want to do analysis you will have to agree to live psychically and in relationship with a very specific person for a very long time, and thus put and maintain a share of libido and affective investment in her" (we don't really say it that way but it is a fact, the patient perceives it right away); at this point many people who would absolutely need analysis, take a step back, if not two. They invoke circumstances of reality (sometimes not even those), and they retreat in horror at the idea of an interdependence with the object to which they are neither trained nor accustomed, indeed, which they feel they must dodge and prevent in order to avoid the pain of possible loss.

This aspect didn't always exist: patients, with a few exceptions, accepted the intensive treatment and the long-term perspective with a sense of relief, because they were welcomed by someone who would seriously care for them with a stable bond.

That bond today is experienced as a threat.

LN: It portrays today's society as an era in which rigid containers and parental equivalents are in crisis: small towns or neighbourhood networks, extended families, the church, mass political parties, and businesses that took in the newly matured child and accompanied him or her to retirement are realities of the past, or nearly so.

There is much more freedom of movement and change: the Bosman ruling[1] has disrupted the reality of football by liberalising the market for players within Europe.

Now, however, there's a crisis of individual identity, where people need others to reassure them all the time, to say "you're doing fine". In all this, a relationship such as that proposed by psychoanalysis seems a gamble, because it requires a very strong trust on the part of patients who are instead inherently lacking in it. To accept from the outset the regulations of analysis (the frequency and fixed hours, the breaks set by the analyst, the payment for missed sessions) would seem almost like a kind of pre-emptive surrender, or complacency to the other, a complacency perhaps little felt within oneself.

I wonder if, today, the gradual construction of the analytical setting, with long consultations or with later adjustments regarding frequency, for example, by increasing the number of weekly sessions over time, is not a process that permits patients to be more aware of their own choices, and to come to build by degrees a desire for analytic deepening. There is a difference between desiring, over time, the greater closeness between encounters, or instead experiencing high frequency as a prerequisite to which one adheres by obedience.

SB: This is a fascinating and difficult issue, because experience teaches that there are situations that evolve differently.

For example, there are patients who, like the famous fox in *The Little Prince*, need to approach the object a little at a time, the one who offers the psychic equivalent of "something to eat". In those cases, the impression is

---

[1] The Bosman ruling is a measure adopted by the Court of Justice of the European Union in 1995 that allowed for the liberalisation of the transfer of professional football players between clubs belonging to European Union federations, with no more constraints related to the nationality of the player.

that, with patience and appropriate relational movements, one can bring a patient to the desire to intensify the analytic relationship.

In contrast, in other cases, not necessarily more severe, if we offer the patient a two-session start, we risk attending to an adaptation to that situation, which makes it difficult to then increase the frequency to the optimal technical level to achieve deep and lasting changes.

There are patients who get used to using what they have, adapting precisely to the two sessions; some, on the other hand, spontaneously ask for more sessions, others flee at the idea of more sessions as if it is the plague.

We analysts know from experience that from three sessions onwards the work becomes different; usually, with a few occasions or exceptions of patients very gifted with introspective capacities, three sessions is the minimum that is needed to set in motion an authentically experienced analytic regression that is functional to the treatment.

I do not go into the merits of three, four, or five sessions, because, on the one hand, there are people who lie on the couch with different needs and abilities; on the other hand, there are different analysts, who are able to function better in one way or another, and who have internalised certain patterns, certain frequencies that have then become habitual for them. For those that say that in-depth work can only be done with four sessions a week, the fact that French psychoanalysis has been functioning well for many decades mostly at three sessions may make us legitimately doubt this.

Whilst it is true that with four sessions it is easier for the analyst to maintain contact with the innermost depth, we must also admit that there is a great variability of factors and situations, as well as of traditions and methodological school arrangements.

Let us return to the issue of narcissistic arrangement, that is, the fact that from early childhood a subject organises himself to keep the centre of gravity of the relationship more on himself than on the object or halfway between the two, because this is really an important point. We find ourselves, today, encountering more frequently patients who have a strongly narcissistic self-centred setup, either out of fear or fixation* (*Fixierung* in German). The latter is a concept that is less talked about than it used to be, but fixation as a mode of habit, of internal organisation, is a factor as powerful as it is silent, which we now detect in many patients who show an insufficient capacity to tolerate constraint, lack, relational vicissitudes, dependence and interdependence, at least at the beginning of treatment.

LN: Since today the term addiction is almost always associated with unacceptable weakness, let's make a brief parenthesis on the difference between this and interdependence?

SB: Indeed. Dependence is predominantly one-sided; interdependence is mutual and shared. For example, if one wants to play tennis, one is necessarily interdependent, one cannot play alone, and the other is necessary; in fact, it is so, even in the healthy and balanced relationship between two people, in the mother–child relationship and in harmonious couple relationships. But if one is dying of thirst, and the other has water, the dependence is one-sided and total.

LN: Here, earlier you were talking about deep work, and analysts use the word *deep* very often. The adjective has taken on many different meanings, to the point that there are questions about what this depth is: "What is deep?" reads an article (Peltz, 2015) from a few years ago. What does deep mean for Stefano Bolognini?

SB: It could be said that it is what influences or even determines a person's life without that person being knowingly aware of it. Here is the first Freudian topic*, which recognises in the psyche a surface level, the consciousness, and the deeper level of the unconscious, with the preconscious intermediate level that I think is actually our main terrain of clinical work, and which, as I will explain later, also comes in handy.

On the technical level, sometimes I find myself in situations where I do not understand what is happening, or what might be developing given the climate of the session; and then it happens that I temporarily retreat into the oldest of psychoanalytic scenarios, which is to stand by and see with patience and curiosity "what pops up", what emerges from the deep.

This is the first topic Freud speaks of: to see what emerges from the most remote cellars or attics, a little at a time; what announces itself in the preconscious, what noises it makes, what signals it sends, until we see what leaks out, perhaps in disguised or incomplete form.

This setup of suspending and listening offers the analyst in difficulty a consistent advantage, which is to relieve at least a little of the initial feeling of operational impotence: when we fail to understand the material or what's happening in the process, the fact that we can be quiet and see what's going to come out is a position, I would say almost a posture, just in military terms, that's very useful because it doesn't rush things. And so, it allows one to see what emerges from deep within, precisely, from the not conscious, or from the not yet expressed, not yet formulated; we can say it in so many ways.

Of course, if an analyst always just kept quiet, waiting, or did not look for other modes of contact and exchange, we would arrive at those paradoxical situations that were talked about in the 1950s, of analysts who did not say a word throughout the treatment and just observed. Today no one would dream of imagining silence and waiting as the only way to do analysis. Yet, in certain sessions when we really can't get a spider out of the hole (an image that effectively depicts the extractive aspect of meaning), the first topical is one of those scenarios that should not be thrown away, because it can allow us not to be too anxious when meaning still escapes.

LN: So, some "negative capacity", as Bion called it? Abiding in a state of uncertainty, without immediately chasing objectivity and reason.

SB: Yes, a state of suspension, of waiting, perhaps frustrating from a narcissistic point of view, but actually natural

CHAPTER 2

Being together

LN: I will now ask you a question that may seem provocative, but it is not, from the point of view of many of our readers. Are so many sessions a week necessary? I'll tell you something that happened to me a few days ago: I was reading the page of a psychoanalytic psychotherapy site, frequented by fellow analysts and psychotherapists from all over the world, who were comparing the depth that can be reached with some patients even in apparently unfavourable situations, for example, by seeing each other once every two weeks. This is an extreme setup for our way of practising analysis; however, it is true that most of us also work at low intensity, with patients at one or two sessions per week.

It seems to me that you pose the question of patient regression as central; is this correct or is there more to it?

SB: We can better understand the question of frequency and regression if we think about extra-analytic affective relationships.

Between one extreme, which is that of casual encounters, and the opposite extreme, which is that of very close cohabitations, almost to the point of symbiosis, there can be a wide variety of modulations of affective rhythms and bonds between people. Returning to analysis, without constant bonding and intense dating there is no experience of what I call "analytic coexistence", which is something more than "analytic cohabitation".

Those who have lived in cohabitation, for example, during college with other students, know that one can live in the same apartment whilst doing each one's own thing, including in the kitchen: one cooks an egg, the other makes a schnitzel, at different times. That is cohabitation. Coexistence is a different thing, in the sense that one is co-interested and involved in the same steps, the same processes, the same relationship in a more intense, more interactive way.

In the case of analytic coexistence, deep aspects come into play, through regression, which very often are precisely those that make it difficult for people to coexist, to live together with someone else even outside of analysis: transference* is activated.

One of the many aspects of analysis is to have the experience of being in two, to do almost a gymnasium of conviviality and to see what happens by being together: what movements, processes, conflicts, pains, what joys or pleasures are created or unravelled.

Those who have a stable couple life know how complete true coexistence and interdependence are, inevitably characterised by sunny days and stormy days: such is relationship life. Moreover, it is difficult if not impossible, in cohabitation, to keep intact the narcissistic images of self and other, tested by everyday life: "No one is a hero to his own valet", said George Bernard Shaw.

Yet, outside of actual cohabitation, no real verification of the relationship would be possible: if two lovers see each other once a week or once a fortnight, at selected moments of high passionate intensity, their encounters may be exciting and enriching, may take on significant importance, and bring out a number of vital and exciting personal aspects, at least for a time; but it is not the same as an integrated and real relationship, because the commitment to an interdependence based on daily cohabitation is much greater, and it is there that—for better or for worse—putting into play all parts of the self and not just those selected narcissistically, a deep and complex experience is realised.

In this, there are substantial similarities with the analytic experience.

A final observation, on the "undercurrents" that link analysis and life outside analysis: we are accustomed—and we are not so surprised—to the fact that, during an analytic treatment, people who do not have a stable relationship with someone outside the analysis, if they do not fixate too much on the relationship with the analyst, over time become capable of spending an important part of the libidinal-affective quotas mobilised by the treatment outside the study as well. They encounter, that is, relationships outside the analysis that have several similarities, without their knowing it, with the course of the relationship with the analyst, and that show what internal areas and levels are moving. Usually, the relationships that are created during a treatment turn out to be gradually more liveable than those that were there before.

LN: I was thinking about the issue of interdependence, which you pose as central. I'm reminded of those friends of mine who, when talking about loved ones, say, "I have a friend I see very little, out those times we do, it's as if we met yesterday". I go further: is interdependence so fundamental?

Isn't it possible that, in a world like this where there is more and more contact and less and less marriage, a person doesn't want to get married, a woman doesn't want children, prioritising the relation with the self? That the human being today has less need for others, for interdependence and deep interchanges with others, and still be okay?

SB: He can be fine just the same, of course, if he organises himself this way not out of defence but because it is the mode he prefers even though it is not the only one of which he would be capable. If, on the other hand, he has structured himself this way because he fears a more lasting relationship and does not want to approach it because he is not capable of it, and therefore cannot, then it is not the same thing.

In short, if it is a true choice, then yes it can be a novelty in this age of ours.

However, it is difficult and risky to make absolute value or meaning judgements: some people want to avoid the risk of conventional and imitative conformism, having to frame themselves according to a certain label; but it is also true that one can "sell" as a choice or as anti-conformism what is instead generated by a deep fear of binding oneself more; so it is good to evaluate from case to case. In certain situations one recognises in the patient the defensive setup of the "fox and grapes" type: the person tells himself, with a kind of self-deception, that he does not want something that he feels or fears he cannot obtain, even when he wants it. And by denying his own underlying desire he saves a narcissistic self-image, but loses authenticity.

LN: Psychoanalytic interdependence is not just a form of training to "being together" with others, a kind of premarital course. On the contrary, we know well that analysis provides not only a gymnasium for deep relationships with others, but also, and above all, nourishment for the relationship with oneself. Shall we examine this aspect?

SB: This is a very good objection and I agree with you, it is indeed so. However, the intrapsychic*, that is, the totality of relationships with ourselves, is not so disconnected from the intersubjective* and the interpersonal*, which are the dimensions of relationship with others.

We all know quite harmonious people who live well on their own and others who live well with someone, just as we know some who are absolutely disharmonic who are bad on their own or in a couple. The complexity of discourse should always be preserved.

Internal contact with oneself is essential for a person to live well, and it is one of the factors that can help in a healthy way in deciding to be on one's own or with someone.

How many couples' lives are based on not knowing how to be alone, or on the need to undo one's own parts by projecting them onto the other, from which one then in a masochistic* way cannot detach oneself? How many people, on the other hand, live quite well with themselves, having, however, had to get used to this regime more because they are afraid of relationships? In short, there is a manifold variety of situations that should be known and focused on a case-by-case basis.

LN: You told us about couples whose members dispose of parts of themselves by projecting them onto each other, and then, in order to deal with each other, form an unbreakable sadomasochistic bond. This strikes me as a most interesting phenomenon, and I'm afraid quite frequent. Can you give us some examples of this?

SB: We are talking about couples seemingly in constant conflict, precisely playing a game that relies heavily on the projection* onto the other of their own aspects and their own internal objectives.

I am thinking of example of an emblematic couple for Italians: "Casa Vianello", that sort of serialised comedy with Raimondo Vianello and Sandra Mondaini that ran for a long time on national television networks, with high ratings.

Italians were amused for decades to watch this married couple with their interminable and above all predictable disputes, because the characters of both people were well known. It was amusing to see how each of them disposed of something of themselves and their inner world, charging it onto the other: this allowed each of them to be themselves in certain respects and to dodge other parts of themselves. When this mix of cross-projections is produced, the distinction between one and the other fades into symbiosis, so much so that the moment one of the two actors died, so did the other shortly thereafter.

Years ago, an undertaker well-informed (not with disinterest …) on industry statistics told me that in long-term couples, the death of one follows the demise of the other by an average of one year, which gives an idea of the depth of the symbiotic development that unites them.

The topic of interdependence is, moreover, a very sensitive one because it runs the risk of immediately slipping into ideology. There are those who think it would be desirable—or for some even their duty—to live in an interdependent couple, whilst there are people who are very harmonious precisely when they are alone.

I think of certain singles (there are some known to all, in very diverse sociocultural backgrounds) who are happily self-centred. Some are capable of relationship, but they do not intend to really tie themselves to another for life: they have had relationships, even important ones, but who knows if they would be willing to go through that contractual step that today has replaced marriage in many cases, namely a joint mortgage, which is not exactly sacred, but in fact far more binding than the wedding ceremony?

LN: A joint mortgage and marriage are some of the great passages of relationship life. Today's analysis, for those who do it, is another of these very significant passages, in duration and intensity.

It has been a long time since the early decades of the twentieth century, when the experience of psychoanalysis was a plunge on the couch six days out of seven, for so many months, rarely for more than two or three years, and then end. At that time, the suggestion was given to the patient to suspend important life decisions until the end of the analysis, because the subject could have been influenced and almost obnubilated by the power of regression and transference.

Now analyses last four, five, seven, ten years, during which time patients and patients marry, graduate, have children, buy houses, move. Whilst, we were saying, there is less initial investment on the part of some, however, the analyses that work become more intimate relations than many other kinds of unions.

SB: Absolutely.

LN: What are you saying here? Are we not going against the grain? Isn't there some "ideology of togetherness" in such long coexistences? Or does care necessarily need these times? I ask this question because we also need to talk to those outside our practices who ask us to account for these seemingly anachronistic features of ours. Some of my patients, joking but not too joking, wonder if there will be time left to enjoy life after their analysis.

SB: … and to detach from the analyst! Which may defer detaching from parents as well, because analysts end up being parental equivalents on whom one can depend very much and for a very long time. I remember when the example of Woody Allen and his twenty-two to twenty-three years of analysis was in vogue. Many people quoted him, made jokes about it, in convivial situations or even during the session.

Then there was a congress of the Italian Psychoanalytic Society (SPI) during which Paola Golinelli interviewed in a plenary session Bernardo Bertolucci, recipient that year of the Musatti Prize, who said that he had been in analysis for thirty-eight years; moreover, the following year Bertolucci telephoned Paola to inform her that after thirty-nine years he had managed to finish his analysis with satisfaction and gratitude.

His was a *sui generis* analytic history, however, because it had taken place with four different analysts. A first one, in Rome, was very old and had died in the process; the analysis with the second, also in Rome, was interrupted when Bertolucci moved to Paris, where he began working with a third analyst; when this one died, he met the fourth, with whom he concluded treatment.

I used to believe that the length of Bertolucci's analytic journey constituted a world record, but this was not the case. Before he died, the famous neurologist Oliver Sacks, the author of *The Man Who Swapped His Wife for a Hat* and many other successful books, revealed that he had been in analysis for forty-eight years, always with the same analyst.

These are striking examples of long analytic coexistences; one does not know what to say.

Were they symbioses that could not be broken, or—as is well possible—was there real and useful work going on? This we will never know.

LN: Jokingly, we can say that people are afraid of analysis because it is addictive, and they are right ...

SB: I think so. It is easy for something unexpected and perhaps not so much desired by the would-be patient to happen.

LN: At this point, I want to speak to you as a mental health professional who has to take into account the sustainability of treatment pathways. How can a therapy such as analytic therapy, consisting of hundreds or thousands of sessions as in the cases you described, be taken into consideration by national health systems and possible referrers such as psychiatrists, teachers, primary care physicians, if one has not already tried psychoanalysis on oneself?

Without direct experience, how do you ask someone to refer your patient, your student, your child, your family member to an analyst, knowing that they will be faced with many years of analysis, with no guarantee of what he or she will accept, with no assurance that a symbiosis will not be established that is then difficult to split? How much trust do analysts demand from the rest of the world?

SB: This is quite true. Let's say that in many cases (not all), especially with severe patients, family members can still realise the progress or at least the maintenance of a state of better compensation when the patient continues the analysis than when he or she interrupts it. Put another way, there are people who cannot stand on their own feet, and instead with the help of an analyst can lead a liveable life. When, on the other hand, we are talking about neuroses, or personality disorders, or narcissistic pathologies, there the therapeutic work-site has different goals than the maintenance and management of a compensated situation: it is a matter of permanently modifying internal defence devices that turn out to be counterproductive, or of maturing in a more dynamic and convenient way underdeveloped parts, not only containing but arriving at new internal balances, new internal contacts, and an enrichment of the self. At that point, however, the work becomes quite incomprehensible to the uninitiated.

It is quite another thing when a group of analysts together explores clinical material in-depth (one or two sessions presented, word for word, by a colleague of verifiable level and expertise). We then get to see how such colleagues, perhaps starting from quite dissimilar individual theoretical bases, often converge in assessing the processes at work and in giving a sense of validity or otherwise to the work in progress. We see this especially at international conferences, where analytic families and theoretical bases differ. When one focuses on the clinical material, one may disagree with some of the technical choices, but by and large all colleagues are equipped and oriented to perceive the meaning and usefulness of the work being done. I believe I have never heard in those clinical discussion sessions phrases such as "It is useless for this patient to go on with the analytic work".

On the other hand, when similar clinical material is presented to non-specialists, it can also be extremely interesting and convincing, but in some cases its complexity is not grasped. These are those situations in which some would say, for example, that it is all about getting the patient away from the family, or that it is all about administering stronger doses of antipsychotic or anxiolytic, or that it is all about getting the patient to change cities, jobs, or habits: that is, offering those crude suggestions that seem to want to cut with a hatchet something that instead requires a very technical, complex, delicate, and precise intervention, like a Swiss watchmaker. You don't give the classic punch on the television for it to readjust.

Now let's turn the perspective around: how does a patient realise that things in a treatment, analytic or other psychotherapeutic, are not working? How does he find the strength to question such an intimate and unequal relationship? Is there the risk of a suggestion from which it is difficult to escape, of a sterile work that the therapist does not interrupt, not to mention the abuses? Okay, there are the patients who, when things go wrong, just pick up and leave. But how can we help those who are unassertive, who can't cope?

I took care of some patients who had stayed three to four years with psychotherapists from whom they did not feel helped. There was the case of those who poured their personal problems onto the patient, or those who ended up turning the relationship into a rather sterile confidence, and so on.

Just to say one thing: on the subject of separations, especially the summer one, which for many patients is the big annual separation, the consultation requests to somewhat older analysts, such as myself, greatly increase from people who are in analysis with someone else and who come to complain on a one-off basis.

The impression is that the imminence of separation, on the one hand, occasionally disrupts the ongoing relationship between the patient and his or her analyst, and, on the other hand, precisely because of the impetus of these separative, pre-separative, and defensive factors, the separation also makes sayable and communicable to an outside listener (in these cases the senior analyst, a kind of "analytic grandfather" who is asked for an extra-treatment consultation) aspects that have been ill-endured and never communicated to the referring analyst with whom one has been in treatment for some time. It is, in short, a consultation-complaint, a complaint-lamentation (Freud said "*Klagen sind Anklagen*", complaints are complaints) presented to an equivalent of a grandparent against the failures of an absent analyst/parent.

In those cases, the task of the analyst who receives the complaint is to receive it with caution, to explore the situation seriously, and to listen well to what the patient is saying; but also to maintain an appropriate suspension of judgement, because these requests for pre-separative consultations are often symptomatic in themselves; they are in essence a sign of ongoing suffering, which is part of the therapeutic situations.

It is true, however, that sometimes they can also be the expression of a true dissatisfaction, and not of a repetitive and characteristic impatience of the patient, stimulated by the suspension of sessions. Hence great accuracy is needed: in some cases it is clear that one will help the patient to return to his analyst, if one feels with sufficient clarity that a defensive reaction to the separation is taking place, whilst in other cases one will invite him to reflect seriously on the rationale for his complaint, which may have its own substance.

Once again, the analyst making these interpretations should pay respectful consideration, but also caution and exploratory suspension, because these are delicate situations. They are delicate from a deontological point of view, from an exploratory clinical point of view, and also evaluative.

LN: Thinking about the future of analysis: I wonder if one of the goals for progress might not be to imagine, among other things, shorter, faster therapies. Do you think it is possible to shorten the time of analysis? Or am I too, at this moment, voicing resistance to analytic work?

SB: After so many years of work, I have gotten the idea that "there is this and there is that"—there are so many different situations.

Meanwhile, one thing that has emerged in the last ten to fifteen years is the increased frequency of re-analysis or analytic tranches. There are patients who have done an analysis in earnest and have finished it in a way that suited their expectations and possibilities at that time, but at a certain point they come to a further stage in their personal evolution and feel the need to restart and explore new areas, which at that time have become important and unclear to them. These treatments are often not true re-analyses, but are a new part of the journey, they are successive tranches that do not necessarily mean a failure of the preceding work, far from it: they are a further phase.

As for other forms of treatment, even famous and proven analysts seem to be focusing on therapies focused on one particular aspect; Peter Fonagy writes about this in all his work on mentalization*, for example.

I think that many working hypotheses in our field should be considered quite freely and exploratively, and I think the future will depend on so many different situations, even at the psychosocial level. Probably the requests for psychoanalytic help are bound to increase, but economic resources are limited and not everyone will be able to afford real analysis.

The important thing is not to confuse classical treatment and analytic psychotherapy, between what is psychoanalytic (and even good analytic psychotherapy can be) and what is not; keeping in mind, however, that even psychoanalysis has become very diverse within itself.

I am of the opinion, with Wallerstein (1988), that there are many psychoanalyses today. There is an underlying element, regarding the different analytic styles or models, that evokes analogies with the rearing styles and models of human beings: children are reared in even very different ways, with different mindsets, criteria, languages, and family styles in distant countries and cultures, in remote areas of the world, and yet they can grow up more or less the same. If there is a certain underlying internal consistency in the growth environment, if there is harmony and authentic introjection of a certain educational model, experienced at the time by the parents, this can lead to a fairly good integration in their relationship with their children, and thus in the children's relationship with themselves. Similarly, we can imagine that, in analysis, the way analysts work may or may not favour certain developments, evolutions, and integrations.

Here we enter a very particular field, which is that of the harmony of internal object relations in individuals, and in analytic schools: children reared in India, New York, or Tuscany may grow up equally more or less well, with a good or less good level of integration and harmony in object relations: the outcomes depends above all on the quality of the internal relations of the parents with themselves as individuals, with each other as a couple, and with each other and their children, in an unceasing and often unconscionable intergenerational chain. It can be said that in many cases families pass on highly characterised and recurring atmospheres and forms of relationships within themselves, which are affected more by these internal components than by the sociocultural or linguistic factors of the extended community to which they nevertheless belong.

LN: We have talked about how difficult it can be for patients to find the necessary confidence to lie down on the couch, and about the very long duration of the journey. Now I can't help but ask you: what for you is the most precious gift that a good analysis gives?

SB: As so many others before me have already said, there are at least two precious gifts. The first is the recovery of a capacity for good internal contact with oneself; the second, which is related to the first, is the improved ability to relate to the other. The two go together. You do not have a good relationship with the other if you do not have a good enough relationship with yourself, and vice versa.

Analysis, when it works well or at least well enough, allows this resumption of good contact. It supposes that after a sufficiently successful analysis not only does a person know himself better, but he understands better many aspects of his own way of being and relating to others. Of course, the knowledge factor is very important, the Central

Ego becomes more aware, but the change does not consist only in this: there is also a better ability to live with and contact with self and others that goes beyond the cognitive factor.

By the way, it is not just about recovering something that has been lost, sometimes it is really about creating from scratch something that was never there.

LN: In your way of doing analysis, what space does fun have?

SB: It has as much space as it can have. There are situations in which you really have fun because the person, without being manic, is in a moment of creativity or good disposition to exchange, to play with symbols and metaphors, and also in a good mood.

Trying to have fun when the patient is sick and unable to do so is not good for the analysis. I believe that amusement is such only when it is true. That then there is a certain fun in being able to be creative is also right, but there is something out of tune with the expectation to be creative all the time.

In many sessions, with certain patients, being creative divides a vain expectation: one has to go through a minefield, or one full of nettles and concealed sharp objects, and having fun would be difficult. One will have more fun when one has worked and reclaimed that field. In some cases a certain creativity of the analyst can be exported in contact with an entrenched patient, it can even be absorbed by him and become interpsychic*; but one should not think that it is established *ex-officio*, to the point of deriving from that a real method.

For my own part, therefore, it depends on the situation. I have had a lot of fun with certain patients, much less or not at all with others; and then it also depends on the stages*. Towards the end of the analysis, with some exceptions, it is more frequent and easier that we can have fun, that we can even laugh together in a healthy way, not excited, not gassed, but just because the potentially funny aspects of situations are grasped in an authentic and shared way.

LN: Let's talk about the end. When you close the door after saying goodbye to a patient for the last session of an analysis, what kind of thoughts do you have?

SB: Thinking back to the various patients with whom I have ended treatments, I note sometimes substantial differences.

One patient complained for some years that despite my attempts to understand her—which she recognised as authentic—she did not feel I was able to nourish her with what she needed, and she mentioned, as an equivalent to the special food I should provide her with to make her well, certain very special bamboo leaves that are the only possible nourishment for pandas.

The patient wanted to stop the analysis, and I ended up with bitterness and a strong sense of concern for her, because I knew she would never find the bamboo leaves. It goes without saying that even from the point of view of narcissism or the analyst's normal satisfaction, it was certainly not a good conclusion to the work: the feeling I had was that I had not been helpful to that person, repeating in all likelihood an archaic failure in her object relationship, whose script I had not been able to change.

With other people, on the other hand, I felt an entirely different sorrow, a healthy grief, such as when my children left home. I felt that I was losing a person who was part of my life, part of my inner world, and I felt a mixture of contentment for her future, for the work we did together, and a veil of sadness because she would no longer come to work with me. It was a detachment, almost certainly a farewell.

I have a hard time tracking down instances in which I felt relieved of a burden. Even a patient who used to attack me a lot, in the sense that he criticised me almost all the time, and who had a prickly, biting temper, missed me afterwards, for a time. When he contacted me again several years later I was pleased, because all in all I had become more experienced, I knew better how to take it, and in many ways I even liked him.

LN: If there is a patient we don't like at all, we have to find even a small part in him that we don't dislike and there pitch our tent. So said Glauco Carloni, one of the pioneers of psychoanalysis in Bologna and throughout our area.

SB: It is a good strategy, assuming that we can really find at least one micro-area that is libidinally viable and possibly expandable: on that basis it is easier to do the work when we can create some coexistence.

LN: Treatises and articles have been written about the conclusion of analysis, and I bet half of the readers right now are wondering, "When does the analysis end? Who decides that? And what happens? How do you figure it out?"

SB: Huge theme. During an informal conversation, Egon Molinari, my analyst, had formulated the rather playful hypothesis that in every treatment there comes a time when, on the scales, the weight of the costs and sacrifices of the investment begins to be less … No, the opposite! It begins to be greater than the weight of the benefit. So, a little at a time, both—I would say primarily the patient, but also the analyst—feel that they should end treatment, as it is no longer beneficial; instead it continues as difficulties of separation arise.

Of course, we are familiar with all those situations, during an analysis, in which the patient says that the work is finished when in fact it is an "escape into healing", a pseudo-healing. These are situations that often manifest themselves after the aforementioned summer separation: for example, the person shows up euphoric at the resumption of sessions; they have discovered that they "feel great" and therefore have no need for the analyst.

These are situations in which there is, in reaction, more resistance than usual: in fact, the patient is angry because the analyst was not there. This is a great classic, known to all analysts, a circumstance in which it is often helpful to say, "Well! This feeling is an interesting development … Let's see if in three months it is confirmed". If, as is often the case, it is a reaction to the separation, then within a month, two at most, the sensation is diluted and the patient no longer wants to terminate: he had put in place a reactive defence to stop feeling the suffering felt during the separation.

Instead, there are situations in which both members of the couple manage to feel that the patient is really better off and has sufficiently changed, has transformed certain ways of being with themselves, with each other, and towards the events of life. At that point, without claiming miracles or imposing changes, the patient feels that the costs begin to outweigh the benefits, and then the analyst explores with him or her the real possibility of saying goodbye.

We also know how, once a termination date is established, sometime later (not immediately, but on average within three months) separation anxieties arise. If the work that has been done up to that point has been substantial, these deep anxieties can be expressed, contained, processed, and scaled-down as a sign of the fear of separation, and they do not invalidate the perception that by now the most has been done.

I describe these scenarios because they are fairly typical, although not valid for all cases.

LN: I thought I would not erase your slip of the tongue "the burden of the costs and sacrifices of investing begins to be less … No, the opposite". I think it has a meaning, which is that when you begin to be able to enjoy analysis and life it means that analysis is moving towards its end.

SB: This is true. There are some analyses that are a pity to end: it would be pleasant to go on, to work again together with that person with whom you have come to understand each other and with whom you have established a good psychological familiarity. But life has its own times and rhythms, and it is right for each person to follow his or her own path.

It is indeed bizarre that the fate of us analysts is that we have to leave the relationship with a patient just when it becomes most enjoyable.

LN: First, instead, we have to go through so many and such sufferances, bitterness, trauma, that many people wonder how an analyst does not take it all home with them. They would turn pale if they knew that we take it home, all right. The real question is, how do we live with it?

SB: Good question. One factor that intervenes in many professions, and especially in those close to trauma, is the development of a certain capacity for functional splitting* in order to enable effective technical operation. None of us would wish that while a surgeon is incising a patient's body they are fully in touch with their mirror neurons and imaging feeling the cut with the scalpel. Does this happen to analysts?

Do we split?

The countless studies on the analyst's countertransference*, understood as a potential hindrance or vice versa as a proactive factor for understanding the other, show that in any case the analyst cannot delude himself or herself into keeping immune from a certain degree of resonance* and emotional identification with the patient.

And whilst an analyst who is completely identified with the patient would most likely lose his or her capacity to think articulately, complexly, technically, and reflectively about what is happening in session, the claim to maintain himself or herself in a detached and neutrally observant condition is simply unrealistic.

These two extreme positions can be represented as "the empathist analyst" (not empathic) and "the apathetic analyst".

Most analysts practice, over time, the maintenance of a measured subjective resonance useful for understanding, and at the same time a parallel level of thinking ability not totally identified with the patient; thus, we are talking about an arctic, not split, mode in the analyst's participation.

Over the years one also learns to work a lot, but not beyond a certain limit.

In this regard, I want to mention an experience that really struck me. Three years ago, I was invited to a congress of veterinarians and pet therapists to offer an analytical perspective on some common issues.

I learned many things, including the fact that the dogs used to treat severely psychotic patients in pet therapy—usually labradors, who do nothing special except be themselves and interact with patients—can sustain no more than two contact sessions a day, otherwise they get sick.

The experimenters realised this by examining the haematochemical parameters of these animals after subjecting them—for a fairly prolonged period—to exposure with severe patients for one hour a day, for two hours, or for several hours a day.

This is a fact that should give us analysts pause for thought as well, because although we have processing, psycho-digestive, and even defensive apparatuses superior to those of dogs, we too suffer at the end of our working day from an overload of projections and projective identifications, and an emptying of energy.

So yes, our work can sometimes lead us to emotional exhaustion, and require us to take long restorative vacations, or at least periods of non-work.

We do not physically move, we stand still, but we are exposed to intensive interaction with our patients.

Most people not in the field, when they hear what kind of work we do or what kind of patients we treat, take not one, but two steps back! And they have a point. Thanks to training, we have more tools, but we still feel the fatigue and have to put a lot of effort into it.

LN: Let me make a conceptual aside. You were talking about a "functional splitting" or sometimes we hear about "functional dissociation*", terms that are often confused with each other.

SB: This is really very difficult theoretical ground, although those two expressions are often used casually.

There are splits of the subject (in this case, of the analyst at work) or of the object (the patient). Here we are talking about a partial cleavage within the analyst, a functional cleavage useful for doing this work, achievable through a series of progressive and modulated dissociative micro-operations, which end up structuring into a fairly stable internal cleavage arrangement: one part of the analyst (the working self) experiences the experiences of the patient or his or her internal objects, whilst another part of the analyst himself or herself (the working ego) performs more conscious and methodical functions of exploratory reflection on these experiences. The ego is the part that thinks about the experience of the self. In the best case, the analyst is not so dissociated and split as to lose a sense of personal Self; for goodness sake, that is maintained; however, the fielding of parts of us that are "technical", selected, and in some ways trained for the purpose, in the long run procures an appropriate level of functional cleavage, which is organised into a specialised identity, a professional Self for work.

It is inevitable that this will be achieved by some dissociation, yes: but it must be seen to what degree.

There are certainly people who pathologically disassociate themselves from doing this work, in the sense that they lose touch with their true selves, replacing them alone with an unrealistically idealising and idealised* self-image (e.g. those of the omnipotent "I will save you" type).

Others, perhaps better trained, dissociate just enough to work without becoming too detached from the rest of themselves: between off and on, between being completely detached or instead fully integrated and in touch, there are many intermediate variations.

During certain particularly traumatic or stressful treatments, it can happen that the life preserver is triggered and one goes off, that there is a true dissociation of which the subject is not at all aware. This can happen; it is part of those circumstances in which it happens that very strong countertransference enactments* blow up the integration.

In contrast, an analyst in good condition does more or less what a strange comic-book character did seventy years ago, called Tiramolla: he was an elastic, simply drawn creature who was able to extend certain parts of his body. For example, it held its feet, its centre of gravity, and the crotch of its trousers inside a room, and meanwhile it stretched out the window with the rest of its body, until it reached the nearby balcony or even the street, without dissociating. It stretched, it protruded, it extended its usual appearance. I don't know if I'm rendering the idea, but I believe that the analyst often manages to organise a good combination of work-ego and work-self, not dissociated from each other: in that case he is neither empathic nor apathetic, and even under very difficult conditions he can modulate himself to reach out to the patient and really contact him ("feel with the patient"), without losing the ability to reflect ("think about the patient").

CHAPTER 3

Narcissus on the couch

LN: From the everyday issues of the analyst we move on to the relationship of psychoanalysis with today's patients. If we go back to our theories, thought arises from the frustration of desire, from expectation. We were talking earlier about the importance of experiencing the absence of the object: mother goes into the next room, then goes out to work, and the child learns to tolerate the separation from the external object-mother by building a good internal object, a thought capable of consoling him. This is the basis of the future ability to be alone with oneself without feeling abandoned.

What do we make of it, if the new generations, and even ours, have begun to function with a continuous illusion of presence? And what about narcissistic overinvestment in self?

SB: True, this illusion is increasingly present.

Usually narcissistic overinvestment in oneself operates when the subject is in the company of the other: then he disinvests him, boycotts him, defensively withdrawing libido* and interest in himself. But if he or she is alone, this kind of person goes into crisis, and needs to delude himself or herself into thinking that he or she has the object there, even if it is not true.

LN: I think of the teenagers who tell me that they can't study because they get hundreds of text messages in the afternoon. Research some time ago claimed that a person checks his phone screen on average every six minutes. For years, there have been help groups and therapists who take care of smartphone addictions.

I wonder if we are at the dawn of a radical transformation of psychic functioning regarding the dialectic of presence and absence of the other, or if the internal transformations are less massive than they seem in the face of such behavioural phenomena.

SB: I believe that this transformation is indeed taking place, thanks in part to (and because of) technology.

Of course, it used to be possible to achieve similar results even without technology: many hallucinated* what was not there, to make sure that it was there.

Without wishing to be offensive to those with religious faith, I believe that many apparitions of Our Lady have been the equivalent, for lonely people who were feeling very abandoned, of what happens in the cartoons of "The Seventh Puzzle" when the explorer in the desert who is dying of thirst sees the mirage of a bar with ice-cold drinks.

We know that one of the basic needs of human beings is precisely that the object be there, perhaps even with the characteristics we would like it to have; otherwise, it can be hallucinated at various levels by our minds.

I think a great transformation, a major psychosocial change occurred with television, in front of which children were placed for many hours a day. I speak specifically, with regard to our country, of television from the 1980s onward, because before that it had exceedingly limited hours.

Thereafter, the endless Japanese cartoons and programmes of all genres and at all hours offered, in a continuous flow, the illusory presence of "something", which allowed parents to leave the little ones in the company of the screen indefinitely, without caring too much. Our colleague Marco Mastella, an expert in child analysis, described the striking case of a 3-year-old boy, whom he saw in consultation, hugging the television set and kissing it as a real substitute for his mother. Then after television came Walkmans, PlayStations, mobile phones. Now the people you see on the street are largely attached to a mobile phone or to some other telematic device.

Never alone. Never without. Never us.

LN: For some time now I have been paying attention to sensory hyperstimulation. When I look at my dog and depict what he does during the day, the stimuli he receives, I realise that it is a few things. For the past few years I have become friends with a calligrapher, a man who has changed his life and now writes on parchment recovering the ancient styles of writing. He, of all people, was making me reflect on how much time was spent in past centuries to write a personal or business letter.

The comparison with the exponential acceleration of incoming and outgoing stimuli and communications offered (and sometimes imposed) by technology is impossible. Meetings, contacts, news twenty-four hours a day, uninterrupted stimulation. Social feeds and feeds on continuous contributions that follow individuals in and out of the home.

I am pondering how much time is left for the emotional digestion of stimuli, or whether conversely we are not faced with an overload of indigestible situations, what Bion called beta elements, raw sensory data that cannot be processed as such, which impoverishes our thinking and makes it fatigued, always under pressure.

SB: Continuous contact at a distance is a way to escape from the self, to take attention away from one's internal experiences: to look or feel outside in order not to look or feel inside. I think—I know that in many cases it is an escape from reality and a resistance with respect to contact with the inner world.

Then, for goodness sake, the practical advantages offered by this hyper-communication are obvious; however, if we think about how paroxysmal this has become, it is more than suspicious.

LN: A further problem I am wondering about, in the face of the new modes of communication, concerns the way of being in relationship.

In an article he recently presented in *Psiche,* our colleague Giovanni Foresti (2019), always attentive to the relationship between individuals, groups, and institutions, referred to the effort that the object requires us to make in order to be in relationship. You spoke of the television set as object/babysitter: this does not ask for a relational commitment on the part of the viewer. It is there available, within reach of the remote control. A young colleague, regarding the function of obstruction that the analyst performs, related to me a comment she received during her supervision; "You are very welcoming, but you are a little obstructive". I think he meant that the other, when he is a true other, challenges us: he induces us to carry out continuous operations of rapprochement, of patience, of creating a rhythm between us and him, between presence and absence.

With the narcissistic drift of society he mentioned, with the replacement of parts of reality by virtuality—I think of kids who meet online instead of live—with the on/off, on or off mode of contact, will we not be pushed towards a progressive loss of the ability to be in relationship? I'm thinking of seemingly well-functioning people who avoid answering the phone, for example, but exclusively use SMS, chat, or voice messages, as well as people who carve out niches for themselves online and increasingly give up being in relationship outside. They feel very much in touch, but they are contacts that do not require the same bodily, relational co-involvement of constant affective investment and acceptance of each other's diversity and timing. What are your thoughts on this?

SB: Yes, indeed the object, if one does not confuse it with oneself, as if it were a part of us, implies an unavoidable experience of otherness.

The otherness of the object, of objects in general, is something very graded in subjective experience: that is, the object can be experienced as totally other, too much other (and then it is experienced as an alien), as a little other, therefore a little different from us, or not at all different from us, as "another self".

Cicero, for example, said "*idem velle, idem nolle, hoc est amicitia*" (wanting the same things, rejecting the same things: this is friendship). He thus painted a relationship that we would call narcissistically mirror or twin*, where the other is an object-Self, not a real other.

At the opposite pole, beyond the threshold of tolerable otherness, the other degenerates into an alien: an excessive level of distance that confronts us with an experience of unbearable monstrosity, precisely an alien entity with respect to what we feel we are, and also with respect to what we would bear for the other to be whilst not being identical with us. So, it is really true that the object, if recognised in its separateness and different-ness, does psychic work, makes us toil, sometimes makes us sick, disappoints. We see this in expanded, extreme form in love relationships: in falling in love an illusion of marvellous coincidence between the two, of an enchanted, dreamy condition in which Cicero's phrase comes back good. But then, as the relationship progresses, even the best-assorted copies experience that this is not exactly so and that the other unfortunately—Damn!—is really another! He's really another, he doesn't want the same things, he doesn't refuse the same things that we would like to be experienced and considered in the same way.

Otherness, then, is a frustrating experience in itself, especially after an illusion of perfect coincidence or similarity, and being able to sustain it, this experience, is not at all a given.

We know from studies of very early infancy that the best conditions for the child's relationship with the environment and object to proceed and develop in a healthy way involve that, at the beginning, the maximum adaptation of the infant's caregiver objects is realised, which—let us not forget—comes from the restrained, providential, quiet, and constant intrauterine world: the smaller the child is, the more "right" he is to want the object and the environment to function in the way he has experienced as habitual and necessary.

Then, gradually, administrations of small, tolerable frustrations will be inevitable and necessary, and on and on away, over the years, a recognition of reality in all its aspects: the environment will have to make its otherness felt, otherwise a little dictator incapable of adapting to the natural limits imposed by existence will be raised.

Television and its technological descendants developed, and were successful, in their function as parental substitutes among children partly because they were meeting the pleasure principle, that is, limiting frustrations, beginning with the presence/absence element of the basic object (the mother, once upon a time, or at any rate a known and constant caregiver).

When I was a child, i.e. in the early days of television in Italy in the early 1950s, there was only one channel and one stood by what the curators of that one programme decided, at that precise time, take it or leave it; then in later years came the second channel, then the third, and then private TV. The result was that zapping began to allow people to choose, discard, decide, leave one programme and move on to another.

At that point the subject became the director of a whole fantasy world, which he not only found ready-made, without any need for his own creative effort, but which he could also select according to his tastes. Now we have come to the possibility of television stories in which the same script, recorded in multiple versions, can be bent to different endings following the viewer's preferences.

It is difficult to evaluate the effects of the countless current techno-logical options, they would risk being biased and very coarse; however, the suspicion is that going forward in this way we end up fostering detachment from the real world, facilitating the hallucinatory dimension and substitute fantasies. Whereas reality—the real one—does not offer as many options and does not permit us to choose them in such an omnipotent way; therefore, it is possible that subjects are enticed to retreat into the "refuges of the mind" of which John Steiner (1993) speaks, into self-defined, protected, reserved worlds, in fact non-relational and not connected with real objects and all their otherness.

Needless to hide from us, this is the great autarchic risk that also presides over so many cases of drug addiction and makes so many seemingly "relational" relationships in fact very solipsistic.

After all, many couples stay together without being in a relationship.

LN: In this regard, I tell you two situations, one analytic and one not, then you tell me what you think.

The first is that of Amedeo, a fictitious name, a 30-year-old boy in analysis at two sessions a week for over five years. He doesn't have the drive to have a third weekly session. In a crisis with his studies, scared of work, he stays at home with two depressed parents, resigned to life. He has few friends, few girlfriends. His only glimmer of life lies in the fantasy worlds of video games, within which he spends many hours.

After years of working together, he recognises that not only is he terrorised by the adult world—he experiences the idea of a work contract as a condemnation to slavery that will lead to consumption and death—he is also terrified of emotional relationships and love. He never loved girls; he was in them because he had to. Maybe he had sexual desire, and I say maybe.

We recently talked about *The Truman Show*, Peter Weir's movie with Jim Carrey, and he concluded that maybe he wants to stay in his fictional world, if others don't remind him too often that there's an outside world. I'm thinking of the phenomenon of the hikikomori, which we imported from Japan: kids who live reclusive in their rooms. How difficult and complex is it to work with these people who isolate themselves in their non-life?

SB: The discourse pending between the two or three sessions is significant, in the sense that it is as if he is saying to the object (in this case the analyst or the analysis as a whole), "Dear Object, I am sorry but in you I invest no more than that! The centre of gravity of the line between us I keep retracted toward me, I will not spend, in a deep sense, more than that. I want to stay in my *Truman Show*".

This reference to the movie really makes the point clear. In this case there is precisely the numerical, economic aspect of the relationship (two or three sessions a week?), which is revelatory: the subject (the patient) "quantifies how much he wants to spend of himself" (in a complex sense), at least for now, in the direction of the object, in terms of the number of sessions.

LN: I will take this opportunity to get some free supervision: what to do in these cases? Or what not to do …

SB: Each case is its own story, so I can only fantasise in a very crude manner what I would propose. I have been in situations that are not identical, but quite equivalent.

Often we invoke the fear of the relationship as something that at first prevents the subject from moving from this withdrawn stance. However, this seems to me to be one of those cases in which the subsequent strong fixation to that way of being, a way that is structured over time until it becomes characterological, plays an even greater importance.

That the subject then became fixated with that way of being because he or she originally suffered traumatic situations, fears, or otherwise deterrent experiences with respect to proceeding towards the object, there is no doubt; nothing arises by chance. But the power of fixation, when one settles, organises, and structures oneself in a certain way, can in turn establish a block that resists even the analysis of fears.

In short, a sometimes "feel-good" ambition of the analyst might be to—in certain cases, moreover, entirely appropriate—explore to the bitter end, in an insistent way, the area of obstacles that, on the basis of trauma or fears, oppose this person's exposing himself and spending more time in the relationship with the object.

We have to recognise that, in certain cases, after things have been arranged in a certain way by post-traumatic defence, the subject has ended up being comfortable in this arrangement and does not want to give up the secondary advantages, the benefits, an identity now established on this basis.

In the latter case, I believe that, alongside all the facilitation work that is usually done so that the subject feels comfortable in the relationship and can know the joys of shared creativity, it is also inevitable to confront the patient by speaking at the level of the conscious ego: I would say that by providing him with a "photograph", a conscious representation of his way of being that allows him to see himself (*It vedersi*) and protect himself (*It av-vedersi*); or, if you will, a map that allows him to situate and orient himself cognitively as well. After all, the narcissistic investment in this way of being (as when one says to another, "I'm a king!" or as well: "I'm not the type to do it any other way, I'm made that way, I like to be that way. Take it or leave it!") runs the risk of becoming self-satisfied and very cohesive, such that it prevents development.

In order for a strong cohesive narcissistic fixation not to materialise permanently, one must also "see" the subject with his integrated conscious self, in the presence of all his internal instances, and be able to more consciously represent this aspect and its advantages, so as to reduce the narcissistic glaze that has been produced around his unlimited, highly gratifying sovereignty.

LN: In short, one can show the ruler his fear of losing the imaginary kingdom.

SB: There are people who have created small surreal subjective kingdoms, for example, in a steel platform in the middle of the ocean. Every now and then the newspapers talk about it. In an Apennine valley in Emilia, there was a guy, clearly psychotic, who had hoisted a coloured flag over his house, which was isolated out in the countryside, declaring that he had created a state of his own in which he "minted currency". This individual, in the midst of delirium, had been printing a currency he called "roric" (in a time when we had yet to hear of cryptocurrency!); however, he retained a split, adequate, and fairly preserved part of himself, so he was able to work in a local business, living discretely, in a condition of compensation. His co-workers, as a joke, knowing of this fixation of his, had organised a cruel prank by announcing to him that the paymaster, who paid him his salary at the end of the month would do so in "roric" instead of euros. The subject fiercely objected. As they say: he was quite mad, but he was not stupid

So, this man cultivated a psychotic, autarkic, autonomistic, narcissistically very invested internal area: in his microscopic realm he was a ruler. Still, thanks to the split, he was able to live partly in reality, although he was a very solitary individual outside of work.

LN: So, you argue that work at the level of consciousness, with the ego and on the patient's ego, can help him by causing him to "gas" less, or at least to like himself less in these regressive aspects?

SB: To like himself less, in a sense, yes.

However, I think this is possible with patients who are healthy enough; if a patient is really as I assume the individual I told you about was, then no, there is no ego work, no reasonable commentary that helps. Of course, it is true that the burlesque operation put in place by his colleagues at least allowed those around him to ascertain a certain quota of preserved sanity.

The story I have told you might at first glance call to mind (but we shall see later a substantial difference between the two events) the famous myth of Agamemnon, who sends Palamedes and other Achaeans to pick up Odysseus, on the beach of Ithaca, so that he sails with them to Troy fulfilling the covenant of alliance he had signed with the other Greek kings. Knowing that Odysseus pretends to be insane in order not to go to war, Agamemnon's emissaries subject him to a kind of sanity test.

They find him engaged in an insane act: he is ploughing and seeding salt on the beach. Then, to test his exhibited insanity (on which they evidently harboured legitimate doubts), they place little Telemachus, still in swaddling clothes, in the path of his plough and watch. When Odysseus with his oxen arrives in front of his son, he stops and turns, describing the famous "semicircle of mental health" that Kohut will also discuss in one of his historical works, and goes around the child without killing him. At that point Palamedes and the others pick him up, because they have realised that he is not as crazy as he wants them to believe.

There is an important difference, however, between the two stories: Odysseus was not crazy at all, he pretended to be; the "King of Roriland", on the other hand, was, at least partially so.

LN: You were able to capture the atmosphere of the second story I had in store, because it is a raw story of death and madness. It is about a person I met the only time I entered a prison. He was a young man not even 30 years old, who a few days earlier had tried to hang himself. He had been in prison for a few weeks, because a few months earlier he had killed his 20-year-old girlfriend with several stab wounds. I had an interview with him in a room in the infirmary: I remember him as quiet, tall, and blond, just another guy. He told me that he had been together with this girl for two years when she informed him that she wanted to leave him, "She didn't have to do it," he added, "but I understand that I was wrong. I acted on impulse, when I should have let her think about it for a week or two. Then she would have come back with me", "Or else?", I asked him. "She had to come back with me".

SB: He couldn't even consider a different conclusion …

LN: Exactly. If we are more and more accustomed to a narcissistic object, a narcissistic world with little frustration, the imaginary reign we were talking about earlier, the reaction to frustrations becomes difficult, anguished, violent.

There are, however, frustrations *par excellence*, ageing and death, from which there is no escape … What is the relationship with these eventualities of the people around you, and analysts in particular?

SB: Here we enter a difficult and potentially tragic chapter. Analysts know of the difficult or impossible representation of death for all individuals. Likewise, they know of the anticipatory anguish aroused by experiences of helplessness in the face not only of transience or the passage of time, which can be intellectualised as abstract concepts; but also, more directly felt, though unconscious, to the feeling of loss, along with youth, of a share of vitality, subject to individual differences between subjects.

Usually analysts, thanks to their personal analysis, are aware of and resigned to this. Incidentally, the conscious and responsible representation effort of this painful reality—that we grow old and then die—has been massive, in the last ten to fifteen years, by the analytic community.

The International Psychoanalytical Association (IPA)[2] has established a special international study committee (Committee on Aging) that deals both with the psychological issues of human ageing in general, with its experiences and problems, and, tangentially, with the psychological and professional issues related to the ageing of analysts themselves.

And it is nothing new that analysts, when studying certain phenomena, turn their gaze as much to the external environment as—introspectively and self-critically—to one's internal environment.

Incidentally, as is well known, there is no official age *per se* that prevents one from practising as an analyst; there is, however, a limitation that the various analytic societies state, but do not always strictly follow, regarding the possibility for the senior analyst to perform in an official way the functions of training, i.e. of a didactic nature.

Even in this area, however, it is known that the variability of individual efficiency is remarkable: there are analysts of great quality who manage to remain so until a very advanced age, whilst others decline earlier.

On the possibility of representing to oneself with sufficient, resigned, and depressive realism (depressive in a good sense, in the Kleinian sense, that is, of sad acceptance of reality even in its unpleasant aspects for the self) the evolutionary arc of the person and of the analytic profession, also with reference to the guarantees of adequate standards of functioning in relation to age, the international scientific community has moved: it has at least begun to highlight the problem, to study it in depth, to produce work on the subject, which deserves recognition.

---

[2] An international association founded by Sigmund Freud in 1910, today it encompasses all the scientific societies in the world that identify with the Freudian tradition and share a demanding training model. There are about 12,000 IPA members worldwide, and 5,000 trainees in training. With its three continental federations, it is present in sixty-seven countries. For more information, see the official website www.ipa.world

A realistic, depressive stance of acknowledgement allows one to better tolerate the loss of omnipotence and therefore the experience of partial helplessness that the human condition inevitably entails from a certain point on. One grows old, and one must dispose oneself to this, even if one is sorry.

CHAPTER 4

Soul and body

LN: It is the law of the body. A body that man has always tried to modify, for aesthetic, athletic, health reasons, but which remains an inescapable real fact.

Today more than in the past, however, there is the illusion, and in part even the actual possibility, of being able to do without the body in social relations. You spoke of omnipotence, and it is no mystery that one can reconstruct one's identity online through avatars, fictitious profiles, retouched photos. For some individuals who spend a lot of time online, these are just as real self-images as the real thing, if you'll pardon the pun. There is gender fluidity, whereby one can go beyond biological fact in search of a different identity, felt to be more in tune with one's desires and imagination. There is the issue of cosmetic surgery, now practised by younger and younger girls and boys, dissatisfied with their own forms. And then relationships are played out so much at a distance, via text.

Even analysts, behind their couches, can illusion themselves at times with a different body, a different age, because of patients' transferential fantasies, to which they are exposed for many hours each day.

If the body is left aside so much, if there are fewer opportunities for integration between identity and somatic data, what happens to our relationship with corporeality?

SB: The relationship with the body can be denied—or even denigrated through outright denial*—when a person refuses to identify with his or her own bodily reality and imagines that he or she is who-knows-what, or who-knows-who, or who-knows-how, disallowing the evidence of what we are.

In this last historical period we have witnessed a great investment in the body, a narcissistic investment that has various origins.

Yesterday, I took my car to the car wash, and I had to wait an hour before collecting it. I didn't have time to walk home, so I wandered around the neighbourhood, in the first suburbs, and I was surprised with the enormous number of places dedicated to personal care: in addition to the hairdressers, gyms, and parapharmacies, I found an incredible number of tattoo parlours, stores dedicated to nail care, along with the flourishing of smartphone resellers and mobile phone repairers, but these devices are already more relational prosthetic tools, albeit at a distance.

This finding makes me think of an overall withdrawal of libido about oneself and one's body, most likely replacing a similar share of object investment.

It is the argument we were making earlier: along the axis that conjuncts the subject to the object, the centre of gravity today is somewhat withdrawn towards the subject, in a narcissistic form. There is an increased care for one's bodily self, which would not be a bad thing at all if it were not—because of its unexpected proportions—the possible sign of a certain withdrawal from the positive relational tension towards the object, the other-than-oneself.

In other cases, however, we seem to witness an alienating claim of detachment from one's bodily reality in order to represent oneself in a para-hallucinatory way as another, as we are not, as one is not.

We see this, in mild form, in individuals, both men and women, who we might call "die-hards" who act, dress, and behave as if they were still boys. We have witnessed the sometimes baffling and ultimately rather miserable spectacle of political figures, celebrities, champions of irreducibility, who denied evident limits to all but themselves; and in some cases the result was pathetic, to say the least.

In the unassuming everyday, a scene that to me evokes endless sadness is when we come across a family unit carrying around an old man, clearly a grandfather, after equipping him with a baseball cap, the kind with a visor, common in America, to make him witty. For me, the 75-to 80-year-old grandfather, wearing an American boy's cap, constitutes an example of a collective denial of his true nature, age, and status, as well as revealing an obvious loss of respect on the part of his family entourage.

But the list could go on: for example, there are forty-to fifty-somethings who exhibit "boyishness" by dressing themselves as teenagers or in a caricatured way, to free themselves from a parental role model with whom they do not want to identify.

Basically, it is a way of mockingly playing with adulthood, mockingly attacking the equivalent of a paternal object.

LN: Some, listening to this conversation of ours, might object that it is a good way not to grow old.

SB: It is a way of deluding oneself that one is not growing old and that one is not ageing.

LN: And isn't that a good thing?

SB: It depends. If the effect succeeds convincingly, then yes, it means that the look is set up in an authentically playful way that allows one to self-represent oneself even so with a good level of awareness and all-in-all harmony.

If, on the other hand, one perceives some jarring, or stereotyping, as is the case in many instances, the impression is that there is a strenuous attempt to falsify one's identity and real age.

LN: There was a time when people couldn't wait to grow up, whereas now there are many people who not only don't want to grow old, but often don't even want to become adults. I was telling you about patient Amedeo, but I also have a host of friends, male and female, who don't think about getting married at all.

Is it so essential to become an adult? Isn't the age enough? Is it not possible to remain young inside as long as one can?

SB: As I said, some succeed in a fairly harmonious and all-in-all pleasant way: they present traits of authentic playfulness that harken back to when one was a child or teenager. And this is a good quality, if it does not prevent access to the area of responsibility: responsibility is a characteristic of the adult person. There are those who manage to admirably reconcile the two qualities, that is, they remain capable of playfulness whilst also becoming capable of responsibility. In many cases, however, the two dimensions are split, and the subject definitely tends to dodge responsibility. In those cases the impression is that basically "the horse rejects the obstacle", that is, the person denies reality.

With respect to the body, there is another issue that is very close to my heart, because I spent my psychoanalytic training years in a general hospital and worked a lot on psychosomatics*. Today we are seeing a real epidemic of autoimmune and rheumatological diseases, even terrible ones like sclerosis or scleroderma. Breast cancers affect even very young women. Gastritis and colon disease are widespread, and then childhood diabetes, cardiovascular disease, and the list could go on.

At the same time in the common vernacular, psychosomatics are often regarded as the same as an imaginary ("You don't have anything, it's psychosomatic"), or as a self-defeating arrangement ("You give yourself an illness"), as if to emphasise a masochistic will. Even among fellow psychotherapists, and even analysts, there are those who still tend to interpret illnesses somewhat mechanically as symbols, on a par with hysterical conversion symptoms. Perhaps gastritis is the outcome of something we cannot digest, or psoriasis on the hands a symptom of avoidance ("Who knows what it is that he won't allow us to touch").

If you listen carefully to the stories of psychosomatic patients, you happen to find traumatic events, unexpressed emotions, unliveable situations and relationships. I think we would do meritorious work in devoting a few words to contemporary psychoanalytic thinking on psychosomatics.

And yes, maintaining a sense of complexity, obscurity, and primitiveness in these processes is necessary, because it is all too easy to find "interpreters" who express themselves with excessive self-righteousness in the gratuitous and often aggressive manner that you mentioned. We know how defensive it can be to simplify and trivialise this kind of complexity by resorting to wild interpretations.

A great deal has been written on psychosomatics, particularly by the French and Argentine schools.

A constant and interesting feature of their investigations is the clinical focus on individual cases, with their innumerable specificities and declinations.

Difficult, on the other hand, to draw up a convincing general treatise on psychosomatics, as was once attempted in the example of Alexander's (1950). Attempting to identify a clear consequentiality between somatic diseases and certain deep meanings or configurations (gastritis signifies such-and-such, kidney stones such-and-such ...), risks in fact giving room to unrealistic and oversimplifying hypotheses, and to somewhat forced theses.

Conversely, individual histories are often complex, and their exploration (whether biographical or as session material) almost always allows for enlightening openings; concepts such as that of insufficient representational capacity, i.e. poor ability to think about and depict certain internal psychic events and processes in an imaginable way, or that of an introverted attack that the subject ends up turning against himself or herself, are worthy of enormous attention for us analysts.

Personally, I believe that we cannot yet trace true general patterns in the psychosomatic field, except by referring to basal defects of mentalization.

I have come to realise, however, after reading many valuable contributions, that today's psychoanalysts enter the subject matter in a truly analytic way, that is, exploring, suspending, connecting where it is possible and sensible to do so, but with realistic theoretical prudence. That there is a general sense in many of these vicissitudes that then unfortunately become vicissitudes, can well be assumed, on the basis of both the more or less traumatic histories, and the type of object relations profused in each individual. However, a certain caution in conclusions is always advisable, especially since we are talking about a field in which it is easy to "catch fireflies for lanterns".

LN: Earlier we talked about object control, hyperstimulation, and pain avoidance. It seems that depressive feelings are kept out of consciousness by sensory control and stimulation, which allow the engine to stay revved up. If the twentieth century was occupied by the dark evil, depression, I wonder and ask you if the twenty-first century is not the century of anxiety disorders.

SB: The internal alarm factors have changed. As we said earlier, today we are witnessing a strong shift from discomfort due to excess pressure from the superego to that related to the Ego Ideal, with the result that they are more prevalent feelings of shame and inadequacy than feelings of guilt.

People by and large are much less fearful than they are ashamed; they fear not being adequate and not living up to their standards, and not being attractive. On the other hand, they are less afraid of being guilty of something; in fact, they are ready to claim a thousand reasons to alleviate their own responsibility.

LN: There is another issue I wanted to mention about the hyper-presentation of stimuli and continuous presence. I think we can talk about a dilation of the present whilst there is little room for memory. Little time is spent reminiscing or recounting the past, there are videos, photos, but they fix a moment, and then they are rarely looked back on.

SB: True, images are captured there and then, and then no longer remembered. There is no interest in the past, in remembering, in a three-dimensional view of time.

LN: There is such a richness of the present that even planning is of little interest. On the other hand, if one wants to remain a boy forever, the future is of no interest, life is now. I ask you, this timeless man, what does he do?

SB: He makes great *aperitifs*, many *aperitifs*. We are in the civilisation of Prosecco (which is very pleasant, by the way) and appetisers.

The *aperitif*, as a social ceremony, has the characteristic of being quite exciting, with bubbly, and of not being very demanding—you don't sit in a specific place, next to two or three people who would then be the ones you would necessarily have to talk to during the evening, in the case of dinner—but you keep yourself floating, floating, even from the point of view of contacts.

The *aperitif* promises much, and keeps all possible options open.

It is equivalent, in a sense, to the exciting stages of flirting, of the momentary pleasurable interaction, full of premise and promise, which does not entail (in regard to otherness and frustrations) the loss of the somewhat magical feeling of being able to glide pleasantly over things, enjoying them without binding oneself to them, in a heady whirlwind of contacts and seductions.

It could be said that today's relational style is very congruous to the *aperitif* or *apericena* (as opposed to the far more constraining dinner), in that it offers the possibility of maintaining relational distance and mobility, and of experiencing exciting stimulations, precisely because of this indeterminacy that keeps all the games open.

LN: And in this situation where one helps oneself with bubbles not to feel lack, not to feel pain, to slip into a manic excited state until old age, there is the profession of the analyst. Truly it seems against the grain for a profession that has profoundly dilated, over the past century, the time and cost required for its training. So many persons talk about "analysts", but when we consider IPA psychoanalysts, we are talking about a person who has experienced personal analysis at four sessions a week, often for more than five years, if not six, seven, eight.

SB: You are right, it is not uncommon to be above five years.

LN: It is a very demanding training. There are also the years of supervision, the different models to study and integrate, whilst we are seeing a decrease in patients who require intensive analysis. Some colleagues, in order to continue doing this kind of treatment, at three or four sessions a week, lower their fees substantially.

On the other hand, why then would people invest so much in something that is perceived as fundamentally painful? Moreover, intense addiction such as analytics seems to be no big deal, for today's patients. What is the state of health of the psychoanalytic profession today?

SB: Well, it's hard to say, because the professional title, however unrecognised academically, is coveted by many, and there are many people who use it and display it, even without having received credible institutional validation: so, it would seem to be a title that is still highly valued in an absolute sense. However, if one goes to look at the real volume of professional activity, as has also been done at the official level by some analytic societies, including the Italian Psychoanalytic Society

(SPI),[3] one learns that it would be difficult today for an analyst to live by analysis alone. There are those who do, there are those who succeed; but it is not as easy as it used to be, for all the complex reasons we have hinted at with our previous discourses on autonomism as a value, on the prevailing emotional autarky as a collective ideal model.

Today's culture makes temporary dependence on analysis not only fearful, but socially shameful: "You are in analysis!" is still said in a derogatory way.

Accepting, as you said, an intense dependence seems to be done not only from a deep fear of involvement or attachment to someone else, with a stable object, but also a sense of diminishment, of loss of self-value and self-image.

It is true that psychoanalysis has always worked to empower people to really stand on their own two feet, but it has also taught how to stand together with others and to create meaningful bonds as a couple, or as a family, or as a work group, or otherwise not to be autarkic. To know how to be alone if and when necessary, yes, but not to isolate oneself and be fiercely independent, always and at any cost.

Proposing today a long-lasting, stable, bonded relationship, which is very expensive (though then not so remunerative for the analyst, given the development of today's professions), risks to be very dissuasive given the spirit of the times. When a patient comes seeking help, he or she feels that analysis is an expensive experience, yes, but expensive in every sense: economically, but also in terms of time and energy.

Here, today, many patients do not feel it as a protective proposition, nor even as an opportunity for evolutionary space, personal freedom, and self-work. No: they feel it as a yoke, a constraint, a declaration of powerlessness.

In short, negative experiences, at first impact, can be very strong.

---

[3] In 2004, the SPI completed a thorough survey, repeated in 2014, on the type of work done by its members, and the number of hours worked on a weekly basis in analysis, at three or four set-time sessions, and in analytic psychotherapy, at one or two sessions, respectively. The results testified to a gradual decrease in the frequency of sessions of analytic treatments, and an increase in work in psychotherapy at one weekly meeting. The results can be found online in the Profile of the Italian Psychoanalytic Society in 2014 survey in the section "The Care/Clinic: Who and What We Treat" of the website spiweb.it

Analysts usually have something that other practitioners in the field do not have, namely in-depth personal experience of contact with the inner world. As a result, if they have done all they had to do to become analysts, they realistically know that it takes time and a lot of shared work to deeply change a person.

They know that it is possible to help a person progress if one accepts these assumptions; they know many of the difficulties and travails that analytic work requires (for example, in experiencing separation in an increasingly conscious and vivid way) because they went through it themselves, during their training.

To summarise in a simple formula, many of them have acquired more than others the keys to access the depth of individuals, thanks to a long and careful sharing of intimate thoughts and emotional turbulence, and are willing to go through these stages and difficulties together with their patients. All this creates an undeniable difference between many of the other practitioners in the field and those outside the mental health field who are used to more relational distance.

One of the reasons why I have written a book on psychoanalytic empathy* is because I believe there is a substantial difference between the healthy, normal and physiological, simple and usually monosectorial empathy of people, and the capacity of analysts to resonate and tune in partially and articulately, without total identification with the patient, with the conflicting and structural complexity of another. It is a different thing. Understanding another and being able to put oneself in his or her shoes without losing one's own, and without blending in with him or her, is not at all easy.

Therefore, the patient may feel that the analyst has a different pace, listening, and internal space than his other interlocutors, and this is what a deep part of the patient is looking for: however, this perception also worries him a great deal, precisely because he perceives that in the work shared with the analyst one really risks going inside things, and inside himself.

CHAPTER 5

Tuning in

LN: Whilst devising this work, it occurred to me that you are a dog lover. Dogs relatively care little about what we say, whilst they are surprisingly sensitive to how we approach them and how we attune to them.

So, I wonder and ask you, is it far-fetched to argue that a particular focus of yours is how to tune in to the patient?

SB: No, it is not far-fetched at all, because "how" is becoming almost more important than "what" is exchanged between patient and analyst. The "how" makes it possible to open introjective channels, and thus foster emotional exchanges, or conversely to close these valuable pathways between the interiorities of human beings.

If we have something of value to say, but we say it in a way that causes the inward channels to close, the quality of what we convey is ultimately not so important; that is, it is not important if it does not enter the right manner, if it is not exchanged in the right way.

It is also true that if these inward channels serve to communicate things that have no transformative or nurturing function, then we do a lot of work for nothing. However, it remains a central theme that the "how" is becoming a must in today's psychoanalysis.

LN: We often talk about tuning in, but what does it mean?

SB: To tune in means, according to the perspective I was describing earlier, to perceive the complexity of the conditions of the other and of ourselves, to communicate inward: from the intern of one to the intern of the other, and vice versa, in a psychically coexisting exchange relationship. I deliberately use the term "exchange" because it is not just a matter of establishing contact (in bodily terms, "skin-to-skin"), but precisely of allowing the passage of internal experiences and thoughts of one into the interior of the other; and by "coexistence" I mean experiencing this exchange in a way that is not occasional, but rather quite habitual and continuative, in a regime of good psychic coexistence.

To communicate in this dimension, one must resonate with various parts of the interlocutor, including the too-often underestimated defensive system. Put another way: if we feel that the other person is closed, it is futile for us to insist on offering him or her something that he or she cannot at the moment receive.

LN: In your definition of empathy as a complex phenomenon, you highlighted that attunement is also necessary with the split and dissociated parts, with the Defensive Ego and with the ineludible ambivalence we have towards the object. I wondered if this definition might not be a warning to colleagues, young and old: closeness to the conscious and manifest aspects of the person, which we can understand as sympathy, or compassion, or generic benevolence, is not the ultimate result to be achieved, but only a very partial component of the analytic setup, which instead must also take into account the shadowy areas, sometimes so dimly visible as to seem non-existent.

SB: Yes, after all, being in good sympathy with another person is not that difficult. At least, for many it is not, and in any case that is not where the analytic game is played.

Perceiving, on the other hand, the various transferential and counter-transferential colourings that are not in harmony with good attunement, that is a psychoanalyst's skill.

Many people have developed a refined surface relational dexterity on the basis of which they can establish a pleasant, endearing, or diplomatic relationship with the other; but the true transference to the object may remain hidden for a long time, and initially may escape the perception of others as well as that of the subject himself, unaware of his own true deep currents.

Good technical attunement is by no means the same as "good" attunement; the former aims for harmonious relations whilst the latter results in genuine connection, with positive and negative feelings arising.

Many people not in the field would already be happy to get along with each other; the analyst is in a sense more intriguing and more demanding, in the end even more ambitious. Not that he wishes to argue, but he wants to "hear" the various parts of the other, and of himself with the other, a little at a time, giving time for the mutual defensive system to register, tolerate, and resonate with them.

This is, indeed, an ambitious and frankly specialised task. I would say no more about it at the moment.

It is already rather complicated for non-experienced people to imagine that the analyst is so uncontentious and that, whilst appreciating and duly using the components positive of the encounter, keeps himself cautiously explorative and neutral, suspending as far as possible his own expectations about subsequent developments in the relationship with the patient: experience teaches us that in analysis the emotional "meteorological" time can change rapidly and suddenly. One could say that the analyst is one who, even on a sunny day, considers putting an umbrella in the car.

LN: Today we are talking about how to enter into a relationship with the patient. You have adopted a very suggestive metaphor, which is that of the relational equivalents of physiological exchanges, that is, how people's bodies interpenetrate each other in the various ages of life. Similar to the way a mother can breastfeed a child, or the way an adult can make contact with the body of a sexual partner, so minds can relate to each other. A speech may be experienced as dry, irritating, or conversely it may appear caressing, soft, it may flow smoothly, and so on.

In concrete bodily exchanges, a relevant role is played by mucous membranes, and you have dwelt on this concept a great deal: tell us about the role of psychic mucous membranes in the analytic relationship.

SB: Whereas the skin, which has already been much studied in the psychoanalytic literature, has more to do with external contact, warmth, and support, and thus has special importance as a bodily equivalent in the context of attachment processes, the mucous membranes—which are the tissue of passage between the inside and the outside and vice versa, and can facilitate or impede such passage depending on whether they become moistened or dried out—seem to me to be more specifically dedicated to representing the interchange between the internal worlds. Not coincidentally, they define the most intimate area of relationship that can exist between two human beings.

The psychic equivalents of the mucous membranes are those areas of mind and feeling that have the same property of giving access to the interior and that can facilitate it, consent to it, or prevent it.

We very often feel, when we talk to someone, whether that person is eager to exchange something with us or not. We feel if she is open or if she is closed, if she lets something that we propose to her go into herself with ease, with facility, and and if she proposes to us, with equal effectiveness, something that enters us without tearing our external tissues, passing through the psychic, psycho-emotional channels that are equivalent to the physiological ones, therefore not pathological: without ruptures, effractions, punctures, forcing.

When things are going well enough, the exchanges proceed as in a pleasurable nurturing process, or in a sexual coupling equally desired by both partners, and so on and so forth.

After all, these are things Freud had already anticipated in the *Three Essays on Sexuality* (1905d). He had not said them in this way, but he had laid the groundwork for a theory of psychophysical equivalents.

Many analysts, even contemporary ones, talk about the modalities of mating between minds and whether or not they are fertilising the pathological transpsychic* or the more physiological and natural interpsychic.

LN: This talk of yours brings to mind a note that I read years ago, and which had struck me from a sociological point of view. Speaking of the metaphors by which the psychotherapeutic process is defined, I once stumbled upon an author, I don't remember who she was, who related the increase in recent decades in the number of women in our profession to the prevalence of the metaphor of psychotherapy as a mother–child rapport.

Such a metaphor, she pointed out, would gradually favour a de-sexualisation of the image of the analytic situation, perhaps because, she added, it is easier to have to deal with a patient-child than with a patient-loving-male-adult.

Beyond the considerations that can be made about this admittedly debatable reflection, I wonder if the metaphorical framework you describe, prevalent today, does not risk overshadowing the aspect of peer exchange, between analyst and patient, assimilated to adult sexuality. I wonder if an excessive infantilisation of the patient, who has to take the "analytic milk", does not risk becoming one of those stiffened metaphors that obstruct the development of thought.

So, it seems to me that the concept of psychic mucous membranes revitalises precisely this aspect, because there are mucous membranes in the nipple, in the baby's mouth, but also in the genitals. Does this consideration resonate with you?

SB: Yes, it resonates with me in the sense that there is a need to integrate the various modes of relationship that can be established between patient and analyst. Various colleagues and schools have paid special attention to certain relational configurations: some emphasising a distinctly genital configuration, others a nurturing configuration, others a play configuration when interest is placed in what lies between patient and analyst, somewhat like a toy put in the middle that can be used by both, so we are in the area explored by Winnicott; still others, finally, have studied fusionality more. The area of fusionality, of primitive, skin-to-skin relationship, can be physiological as well as pathological. Recently, so many of us have been dealing with physiological, necessary fusionality. It is the thing that, if it is missed as a child, the adult will unnecessarily seek throughout his or her life, even in improper and unsuitable situations.

The list of modalities and forms in which the analytic relationship can be presented could go on and on: there are situations in which a certain concept stands out in the foreground it could be, for example, internal groups, or the primary scene*, the oedipal triad*, or nutrition, treated by so many authors, such as Melanie Klein, but the list could go on for pages and pages.

For an analyst, perceiving what is the dominant configuration in the relationship that is established with a certain patient is one of the fundamental tasks. Certain patients tend to create an atmosphere associated with a certain scene, and others to other scenes.

Listening to or reading authors who remain a little too focused on a single configuration that in a sense then ends up becoming their speciality, their conceptual workhorse, I am reminded of an episode that happened in a restaurant in Rome, many years ago.

I noticed that the sommelier, who had come in great pomp to our table (there were still very few sommeliers at that time, almost an absolute novelty), recommending a wine that he thought went perfectly with our dishes, had then gone to the neighbouring tables, where the diners had ordered entirely different dishes, to propose the exact same wine. Which had raised doubts and created hilarity at our table: it became clear to us that he had a case of that wine in storage and had to somehow, with great snobbery, "unload" it.

The risk for analysts is somewhat the same: if one becomes a hyper-specialist in the thematics and iconography of the primary scene, or of nursing, or of play, or of mirroring, one risks always selling that same wine whoever is in front of you.

LN: Speaking of fusionality, you mentioned the exchanges between the inner world of one and the inner world of the other, which are fundamental to the development of individuals. Today, however, we live in an era of precarious bonds: everything is fluid, everything is unstable.

Among the virtues I admire about you is that of making people reflect on seemingly simple aspects. Here, in one passage, you write that: "Intimacy facilitates the creation of stable bonds". This strikes me as a pretty interesting and far from obvious consideration.

SB: Yes. When I refer to this, I am referring to integrated intimacy. To speak plainly: there can be great seductors, or great seductresses, who know how to ignite an intentional momentary psychophysical intimacy with a number of other individuals through effective relational arousal techniques. This does not mean that one has built the same relational intimacy, integrated at all levels internally in the person and the other.

Usually, if both affective and sensual and, one might say, cooperative integration in a relational sense is built, a deep and stable bond is generated.

If, conversely, there is a fragility in this internal integration, then yes, it is easy for physical intimacy, affective intimacy, recognition of the bond, and the balanced narcissistic condition that presides over all these relationships to be dissociated: certain people, for example, know how to be passionate towards but not supportive of their partner, or vice versa; others appreciate certain qualities but are ashamed of other characteristics, in a conflicting and sometimes even contradictory way. There are people who would not give up a certain relationship, but do not wish to exhibit it in public because of a kind of supposed narcissistic unpresentability, and so on.

What I mean to say, in much simpler words, is that when you connect quite well with someone at various levels and in various aspects that are not too conflicting with each other, you are more likely to be together with that someone. It is so obvious, it becomes almost trivial, à la Palisse.

LN: I want to ask you a question, at this point, as a corollary. What are the main enemies of intimacy?

SB: We could say that the general psychosocial situation has changed, and psychoanalysis has changed quite a bit, in this regard.

At the beginning of the twentieth century, up to about mid-century, the principal enemies of intimacy were inhibitions, feelings of guilt, persecutory fears, and, in essence, castration anxieties, where castration means many things, including negative judgements of various kinds, declarations of inadequacy, discussions, and so on.

Today, no.

Today, the greatest obstacle to the creation and maintenance of a certain intimacy is given by that narcissistic defensiveness that usually stems, more deeply and far more unconsciously, from anxieties of abandonment.

My thesis, which is rather bold and not very politically correct, as I told you earlier, is that at the root of many of these anxieties today is an insufficient initial fusion phase between infant and mother, which causes the child's relational barycentre to be set back towards the self, rather than towards objects.

Put another way,

> Dear Object, you made me feel bad because you didn't involve me long enough and generously enough in initial physiological fusionality, so you know what I do? I retract the centre of gravity on myself, and to you I allocate a limited share of emotional investment, sufficient to keep the relationship going, but not enough to get me involved beyond my 49 per cent, so that I don't risk getting sick again.

The result of this self-protective setup is that, in their life, individuals are much more careful and guarded about permanently and deeply investing in the object because they must preserve themselves from the pain of separation, abandonment, and lack.

Early detachments from mothers, the rotation of caregiver figures, the precariousness and instability of family units and parental networks, the use and abuse of electronics of human presence … All of these aspects mean that the more narcissistic and more defensive organisation of contemporary subjects makes them inclined not to bond more; and this, by the way, is one of the reasons why, unlike forty years ago, proposing to a patient four weekly *séductions d'emblée*, right away, very often means today that the patient will flee, or say no. Patients often say, "I can go up to one, two …", and this, which is always justified with reasons—for pity's sake, sometimes plausible—on the concrete, economical, and/or organisational level, in my opinion originates from deeper roots, which are precisely what we are talking about. The phrase in which I condense this phenomenon is: "Oh, Object (vocative!), oh, Object, thou shalt not have me: I will put, yes, one foot in the pool, but not two. I will not surrender myself to you, I want to keep control of myself!"

LN: Now I ask you a question that was suggested by your last reflection. You write that just as the primary object—the mother and her substitutes—treated the self, similarly, in adulthood, the ego will tend to treat its own self. That is, the primary relationship serves as a model for the adult's intrapsychic relationships.

If the primary object, in early life, is elusive, precarious, and subject to rotation, as mentioned earlier, how does this type of ego/self-configuration develop in the adult?

SB: It can develop with a similar avoidant, evasive, and elusive mode of the Central Ego in contacting one's Self. Put another way: by identifying with the primary object's relational style, the ego can "specialise" in avoiding contact with the experiences of the Self, repeating intrapsychically what had occurred intersubjectively and interpersonally.

The Central Ego repeats towards the experiential Self the same modes of avoidance, trivialisation, splitting, or what someone else adopted in the beginning, mixing up the needs or experiences of the child's Self.

To give a simple example, when a child is accustomed to a parent who, in a time of need, turns the other way, his or her ego, as an adult, will tend to disregard the experiences of his or her own self, denying or avoiding them. It will turn away from itself, will not take itself into consideration, will be little in touch with itself, and will fundamentally, through identification, transform the passive into the active, inflicting on the self a depriving treatment.

LN: Since you are talking about the different ways in which the ego can work at odds with the self, I ask you a question concerning a very important theoretical-technical issue. You have written that the analyst should not describe the non-functioning ego by telling the patient, "Look at you doing this thing, which doesn't work", because that mortifies, frightens, and creates envy. Rather, the analyst should work on the relationship between the ego and the self, re-contacting, experiencing, and repairing at the level of the self. Is this psychoanalysis?

SB: No, this is not psychoanalysis, just as psychoanalysis is not any of the other theoretical lines that are presented by other colleagues. These are various aspects of psychoanalysis.

Actually, it is not then always true that it is not useful to describe to the patient the specific way his or her ego functions. In some cases it may be useful, so as to help him to portray his own way of functioning. It is, on the other hand, rather useless, in my opinion, when the functioning that would be described is highly pathological, so that the patient cannot change it by good will alone. If a person has hallucinations, it is not by explaining to him that they are not real perceptions that he will be able to stop having them. In that case one would be trying, somewhat forcibly, to dissuade the patient from being as he is, from functioning defensively in a very massive and radical way. Rather, it will be necessary to create internal conditions such that he will recover a non-dissociative condition, which is not an informative-cognitive step. It takes time and a lot of work together. An example of what I am saying is the attempt to signal and describe projections: when the patient says that today we are hostile and projects onto us something that does not correspond to how we feel, but to how the patient experiences at that moment.

Of course, I am not talking about projective identification* that makes us experience what the patient puts in us; there is a big difference. The projection I'm talking about is not something that is put on top, on the outside, and if we immediately communicate to the patient the fact that he is projecting, telling him that he is experiencing us as hostile, in practical terms we are trying to convince him that he is seeing things that are not there, or distorting them.

In cases like this, patients usually get very irritated, sometimes frightened if they give credence to what we say, and feel severely pathological in a way that they know they cannot, there and then, change.

There are other less disturbing situations in which, on the other hand, pointing out the malfunctioning of the ego can make the patient more reflective.

LN: You responded to my tendentious question by emphasising the complexity of psychoanalytic treatment. Today in psychoanalysis there is much talk of transformation, a term that is more widely used than in the past. With respect to treatment, you describe a changing paradigm, using a particular expression, namely, "the transition from crisis to lysis". What does it mean?

SB: We could say that lysis is that process of slow dissolution that little by little changes the characteristics, the consistence, the qualities of a formation, of an internal object, of a relationship, of a characteristic of self or other; crisis, on the other hand, would be a rapid, punctual, concentrated, and inescapable process, a real "reversal" for the previous personality setup, which would allow a completely different meaning to be given to something, a content or a situation, thanks to an apt interpretation, for example.

Lysis has been beautifully described by some authors attentive to developments of the Self, such as our Bologna colleague Alberto Spadoni in his beautiful work "The obscure object of need" (1987), and by many others.

For example, when Heinz Kohut, the founder of the psychology of the Self, describes how formations arise, how they amplify, and then how they deflate and decline the grandiose formations, megalomaniacal aspects, and even archaic idealisations*, speaks of a physiological process that takes place bit by bit, by lysis, if allowed and assisted appropriately by the object. Such a process does not go through an attempt at active conviction of the patient by the analyst at the level of the conscious ego, but rather through appropriate psychic coexistence that facilitates and removes the emergence of these deep formations and accepts phases of mirroring by the subject, necessary to consolidate the sense of self.

Put another way, for Kohut at least some of the grandiosity is bound to be reduced by lysis, to dissolve, if it is given time to emerge and be experienced without premature criticism of the subject.

I object to something specific to this perspective, if one claims to think of it as a panacea, a *passe-partout* valid for every pathology, as it is sometimes presented by the author's more radical heirs.

Many of Kohut's findings are indeed interesting, and I am convinced that in many cases what he claims is essentially true, but in other cases it is not. For example, those, which are not so rare, in which at the origins of the problem there is not a generalised defect in the cohesion of the self, but rather there was a glue, a cohesive element (I call it a "narcissistic glaze") that has caused those areas, those parts, those features of the self, that have been narcissistically invested to harden. The subject then, at a more or less profound level, is secretly proud, proud of those own characteristics, appreciates them and defends them with claws and teeth.

In such cases, in my experience, waiting even years by refraining from interpreting may not be so productive: there is the option originally expressed by Melanie Klein, later taken up by Otto Kernberg, of pointing out to the patient these internal formations, which at their most extreme level lead to destructive narcissism; thus, starting to reduce with active technique the narcissistic element that unconsciously sustains and protects them has more play there.

Sometimes one can grasp without too much difficulty the presence of such a secret, smug pride of the subject regarding those own configurations, modalities or parts of the self, or of one's own internal objects admired for their alleged power; to the point that, if one does not purposefully subject that narcissistic glaze to analysis and "work it" a little, it will always remain so.

To go to the paradoxical, I sometimes fantasise about how the analysis of narcissistically majestic characters might have unfolded. I think of individuals who, until the final collapse, have cultivated the genuine belief that they are the holders of characteristics, qualities, powers superior to those of normal people, perhaps seasoned with a little (quite a bit …!!) of paranoia*: as in the case of Hitler, who had Jewish roots but did not want to acknowledge them, wanted to hide them, and attacked them in others; or in the case of subjects endowed with phenomenal grandiosity, such as that of Napoleon Bonaparte.

I have fun picturing these two characters on an impossible couch and, in reverie, I even go so far as to think which analyst I would send them to: of course, not all of them would go well!

LN: In one of your writings, you argue that "we do not provide cognitive and descriptive information [incidentally, I think you mean that we do not always or often provide it] rather, we exercise the person in the passage of pathways that can bring him or her closer to the 'unconscious'". How does the person practice those passages?

SB: It is true that sometimes we work with our own and the patient's ego, and therefore, at those times, we engage in reconnaissance and descriptive work; however, it is not only, and perhaps not even so much that, psychoanalysis.

I also very much appreciate Ego Psychology—the US theory that was very accurate in its description of the ego and its functioning—has had its reasons and functions, and we can well find, in so many of its aspects, so much so that in my opinion it is unduly undervalued today.

However, the steps that provide access to the experiential area of the self, within the patient and between patient and analyst, are essential. Through the analytic situation we facilitate the patients' contact with themselves, which among other things alarms the subject's Defensive

Ego greatly, often at first: think of the condition of lying relaxed on the couch, for example. Usually, we show appreciation for what the patient is able to bring to the session, in terms of thoughts, associations, dreams, or discourses—which are then also associations, when they are not too superficial and defensive.

However, there are many ways to help a patient discover and use internal channels. For example, a number of colleagues have developed skills, abilities, and I would say really even familiarity with reverie* activity and, therefore, with facilitating similar functioning for the patient when possible.

I emphasise when possible because, if you necessarily want to promote that kind of activity with someone who is not yet able to produce it, in my opinion it does not work, and the attempt may turn out to be a stretch. When, on the other hand, the patient begins to be able to share, experiment, and appreciate that way of proceeding, then yes, the internal enrichment becomes substantial.

More generically, in my view, the preconscious is that cultivable, creative area, within which one can train the other to appreciate attending to the internal world. Let me explain further. I likened it to that part of the sea near the beach, which does not present great abyssal products, but which allows everyone to immerse themselves in tranquillity, to abandon the controlling upright station and to float, allowing themselves to float: which means to associate, to remember, to imagine. This, usually, helps patients get into the water, a little at a time.

One factor that, dosed appropriately, helps patients learn about this dimension and its potential is seeing and feeling how the analyst moves about himself or herself. For example, if the analyst comments very simply: "What you say brings this to my mind", then it shows a liveable way, accessible to all, of valuing what emerges and communicating it to the other.

Of course, we will not necessarily say everything we are thinking; however, through this kind of communication. we make our relationship with the preconscious quite natural and visible, and the patient can, a little at a time, learn to move in a similar way.

If, however, the analyst who is familiar with his or her preconscious exhibits it too much to the patient, the latter will become mortified and shut down. He imagines that the analyst is ranting, and he thinks so defensively, because he actually envies him, in the belief that he will never be able to do as well.

So, just to stay with the sea metaphor, the analyst should not make a spectacular swim at a great distance from the shore; instead, he should do something that the patient, too, can feel as a possible hazard, which he, too, may sooner or later begin to indulge in.

CHAPTER 6

Abysses of the unconscious

LN: I have three questions for you in relation to aspects of preconscious communication in the relationship with the patient. The first one concerns the passage in which you write, "For me, psychoanalysis is not the science of the unconscious, but of the passable way to the unconscious and the natural relationship with it". It seems to me that it has to do with the maritime passage we were talking about in the previous chapter, and it brings me back to what you wrote in your last book *Vital Flows Between Self and Non-Self* (Bolognini, 2019), when you point out that "into the depths of the abyss one goes there by submarine", and, therefore, one does not go there by swimming. At this point I ask you: the unconscious, described in this way, do you see it as a place or a process?

SB: Good question. It could be both, in the sense that the process creates an unconscious that has a kind of topical location. Freud talks about topics, and the *topos* is a place that is actually located in depth. It is true that there are also attics, which are another equivalent in which removed or dissociated contents are stored and accumulated. However, in my opinion, cellars, or the profundity of the sea, more properly render the idea of the unconscious in a topical sense.

The fact that the unconscious is a process is equally true, because the things in the cellar we put there, or our father, or our mother, or grandparents, that is, they derive from something that was "made", in the psychic sense: either because we didn't want to have them around, or because we were afraid of them, or even, as in the case of wine, because they are better preserved in cellars; and in this case there may be an unconscious protective care towards precious design or constituent elements of our Self, which we don't want to put out into the everyday world or which we want to keep in secrecy. Who knows.

This is the case with certain affects, for example, that patients in advanced analysis discover what makes them cry and what they did not know they had inside them. As if certain tears were precious bottles of wine, deposited down in the cellar who knows when and who knows by whom.

LN: Today different psychoanalytic models consider the unconscious in different ways. Other than the Freudian tradition, which you described, colleagues who delve into Wilfred Bion's think of the unconscious as a transformative process of experience. Giuseppe Civitarese (2016), our Pavia colleague who advocates the Bionian field model,[4] says in this regard, "The unconscious is not behind or below, but within the conscious, and it has with the conscious an always mutual relationship of a background figure, which is also on the surface and not only in the depths". I wonder if the central issue is not the passage from considering the unconscious as a place, as in Freudian topical metapsychology*, but to a theory that values the dialectic between consciousness and the unconscious.

SB: I believe that the unconscious is the product of a series of dynamics, no question about that. Such dynamics can be extremely archaic and start from very basic processes, such as avoidance of pain, or transformation from passive to active, the latter being one of the most archaic defence mechanisms. The subject always seeks to be active, not passive; to inflict, not to suffer; to leave, not to be left.

---

[4] The Bionian field model to which I refer is the one developed originally in Pavia by Antonino Ferro and colleagues, which over the past decades has been extended to many areas of the psychoanalytic world. It suggests observing the session as if it were a semantic and emotional field, within which the distinct subjectivities of patient and analyst lose their importance, in favour of shared experience. In it, emotions find signification and narrative through the abilities "to dream" or to do unconscious psychological work that the two are able to deploy. The main function of analysis is thus not to retrieve and describe a removed emotional truth, but to weave a narrative of shared emotional experience, and to help the patient learn the ability to do so autonomously.

Or there is a side-ration away from consciousness. Side-ration means the placement, fixed or dissociated, of unacceptable thoughts or emotions in a sidereal space, much farther than the near and accessible one.

All these are metaphors, of course. It is not that we have to understand them in a concrete sense, as a place buried who knows where. They are abysses or depths, but these words, "deep", "abyssal", are not used at random: metaphorically, they render well the concept of distance from and to the conscious ego, to the Central Ego of the person.

Then, of course, the unconscious lies not only in the basement, but also in the living room, in the kitchen or even in a thoughtful library; and maybe we do not see it precisely because we are too close to the proverbial "elephant in the living room", or because it has fused and camouflaged itself with something else, perhaps—as Professor Giorgio Sacerdoti, one of the pioneers of psychoanalysis in Veneto—by an insidious process of assimilation: becoming similar, to the point of camouflage, can minimise the risks of the other(s) attacking us. Think of all those Middle Eastern countries in which the citizens all wear the same beard or moustache as their leader …

In short, there is an infinite number of possible scenarios, and something may be unconscious whilst being right before our eyes.

LN: The next question I wanted to ask you occurred to me when you talked about the communications to make to the patient. In a passage in one of your books you describe the transition from interpretation to communication, and since I am making you dialogue indirectly with colleagues today, I quote to you a sentence from Thomas Ogden, one of the world's best-known living psychoanalysts, which reads:

I don't find that the term "interpretation" well describes how I speak to patients. I think the phrase "talking with the patient" better captures the feeling of the conversations I have with patients than does the phrase "making an interpretation" (Ogden, 2013).

SB: This is a fascinating topic, on which I would, however, tread carefully.

In this sense: I agree with Ogden that the conversation—as I know him to consider it, that is, in a sense that is anything but superficial or trivialising—has exactly to do with those possibilities of interchange between two people (but also between more than two) that reveal an equivalence with primary interchanges from inside to inside.

A good "conversation" can indeed reach the interior of both inter-locutors; if it is superficial chatter, it reaches no interiority.

The interpretation would seem to indicate, in the best cases, the ability to make new sense of something, which can also happen happily naturally through a conversation, in the deep sense Ogden gives to this term.

It can happen in other ways as well: a famous scene suggestive to me, in this sense, is that of Puss in Boots when he turns the ogre into a mouse and in so doing makes him "embeddable and digestible".

The equivalent of this, in an analytic situation, can be to transform something that the patient experiences as incomprehensible, very dangerous, and not human into something, instead, human, under-standable, and therefore treatable. This is a possible representation of an interpretive process, which reverses the situation and the state of the cat and its owner: in the sense that the cat-preconscious can put the Central Ego-master in a much better condition to deal with that difficulty—or even, somewhat oedipally, to become master of the castle in its place, and also master of itself. In short, it enables him to feel comfortable within himself. This, by the way, would somewhat modify the famous Freudian statement about the ego not being master in its own house: if the Central Ego arms itself with the preconscious, it can be, and it can even enlarge the floor plan of its house!

In cases similar to the one in the fable cited above, however, I am not sure that the term conversation, however familiar, does not turn out to be a bit reductive.

The idea remains valid that the concept of conversation can have a valuable meaning and its own analytical dignity as an indicator of natural fluidity of process; however, in the exchange in session I find there is, perhaps, something more, something more specific that allows us to transform the ogre into a mouse, and thus to recognise an absolutely human nature in something of us that was feared as "dehuman" or superhuman.

I propose another, very common example: there are human feelings execrated for narcissistic reasons. The two feelings that I always mention, because they are feared and detested when attributed, are envy and jealousy: nobody wants to turn out to be, or feel, envious or jealous, because both conditions signal a minus, an absence, something we do not have that the other does. This offends us to no end, so usually people like to proudly claim that they are neither jealous nor envious.

So sometimes I pose with patients in a somewhat provocative way and stage a gag in the session by sentencing, with apparent seriousness, "Yes, it's true, I also divide humans into two categories: there are those who are jealous and envious …" (and, so far, the patient feels confirmed and comforted, because he knows that he will not belong to that miserable category, as he is certainly better than others); then, however, I add "… and they know it" (suspensive pause, which begins to cause some disquiet) "… and those who are jealous and envious exactly like the others … But they don't realise it!"

Through this recitative nonsense, with an intentionally high tone of voice, which somewhat disorients and disrupts the patient's defensive categorisations, I attempt to humanise something that is usually dehumanised, refused, rejected, despised.

Of course, it is clear that there is pathological, deluded jealousy; but there is, also, physiological, normal jealousy; and if this is not there, or rather, if it does not appear (as rejected outside the Ideal Ego), this means that something is wrong.

LN: Earlier you were talking about "it comes to my mind", and now you mention those exchanges between patient and analyst, of conversations and interpretations. In this regard, you write that in psychoanalysis today we no longer consider so much of what happens in the patient's mind as we talk, but rather what happens between him and us. What value can we place on this paradigm shift?

SB: Indeed, it used to be that the intrapsychic was more emphasised, then the interpersonal and the intersubjective were emphasised. Now I think it is time to study more—and I am among those who are trying to do this—the influence of the interpsychic or the intersubjective or the interpersonal on the intrapsychic, and vice versa. In the sense that bidirectional transitions occur between these various dimensions that can change things.

LN: In fact, for some years now, your interest seems to have focused on the unconscious levels of emotional exchange, not always intentional. Let us dwell on the interpsychic, which we have already mentioned and which I think is an elusive and equally intriguing concept.

SB: This concept arises from the observation of modes and levels of functioning in exchanges between people, which in certain situations are not to be considered as true and whole subjects, that is, it is not necessarily the case that the two interacting are so cohesive and so well-defined at the time such an exchange takes place. I'm talking about exchanges at quite healthy levels—I'm not talking about schizophrenia, about people who never manage to remain the least bit cohesive and well-defined.

Instead, I am talking about two people, or rather two human beings—let's keep it broad— who at that moment need neither to define themselves more, as would happen in the interpersonal, nor to keep themselves cohesive in a stable way, as is realised in being "subjects".

In a sense, these are situations very close to instinctivity: the football player who receives a pass and immediately perceives which teammate is better positioned and seems more attuned to him, passes the ball to him without spending so much time perceiving his own subjectivity. I remember a very witty basketball teammate who by proposing a very quick "*dai-e-vai*" (a pass of the ball with a return pass as fast as possible, to disorient the opposing defender) shouted to the closest teammate he engaged in a split second, "UNDERSTAND!!!"

In reality, they were instinctive processes that were no match for the dynamics of a pack of predators on the prowl.

They are those extremely good, happy, and creatively unstructured situations that we can allow ourselves in very special, infrequent conditions, in which we trust ourselves to coalescence with each other or to cooperate psychically, without standing there constantly defining "I am me; you are you".

If you will, these are circumstances in which the *we* is more fusional, but not confused. It is those situations that go back to very early mating between mother and child, where things work without having to establish who is one and who is the other, because a natural cooperation spontaneously comes into operation.

For example: we know that, during sucking, there are moments of great fusion and good bidirectional abandonment between baby and mother, where they cooperate. If the baby did not suck, the mother would not produce milk. The mother takes pleasure in producing milk, the baby takes pleasure in sucking, and at that moment they are a unit, without being confused: they are fused. Confusion is a pathological element; fusionality can be, in the appropriate stages, the element, the aspect, the most natural functioning of the world.

The same can happen within a trio, a quartet, a musical quintet, even an orchestra, in the happiest moments when people play particularly well together and experience non-pathological cooperation: it is not a mass losing its brains, as in the great regressive, pathological masses' upheavals. It is cooperative work, in which one is quite happily fused and functions by composing a whole.

In analysis, this can correspond to situations, as the one described by a Trieste analyst, Savo Spazàl, (1990) forty years ago, who recounted, "At that point the things we were saying to each other could have been from both of us: said by one or said by the other, because we felt them to be true and they were circulating".

It is like the milk between mother and child, or the exchanges in sexuality and other moments of greater freedom and more fusional joy, not confusion.

LN: Does the difference between fusion and confusion have to do with the presence of anguish, or something else?

SB: Yes, it may have to do with anguish, although anguish, in my opinion, is a separate chapter. In fusionality, interpenetrations and interconnections occur in the right bodily and psychic spaces, at the right time, when there is a desire in both for this to happen. This can happen even among several people, as I mentioned in the orchestra example.

Fusion happens when things are working well; confusion, on the other hand, implies an anguished loss of a sense of self or even of the *we*. This was well described by French psychoanalyst Paul-Claude Racamier, an expert on psychosis and the creator of a historic therapeutic community ("La Velotte", in Besançon, an admirable example of a treatment institution that really specialised in the treatment of severe pathologies) when he spoke of the difference between *depersonation* and *depersonalisation*. In *depersonalisation*, which is a pathological phenomenon of the psychotic type, the subject is anguished, he feels that he is losing his integrity. In contrast, in depersonation there is the pleasurable feeling that one is not thinking only of oneself, or for oneself, or with oneself, but with others: a level of fusion that is non-confrontational, non-anxious, non-disruptive, non-schizoid. Regressive, yes, but in its own way physiological.

LN: You replied that anguish is a separate chapter. Shall we open this chapter?

SB: Yes. Anxiety, anguish, and panic, which are the three gradations of feeling anxious, in many pathological situations are not actual feelings: they are tensional states, which often arise precisely when the subject is desperately trying not to feel a feeling. These states usually dissolve when the subject gives in to feeling the feeling. For example, when a patient who had hitherto resisted a warm affective feeling, rejected by him at an unconscious level, finally lets go and starts crying, he no longer feels anguish afterwards. He felt very strong anguish before, when he was tensing up in resistance, because he felt the risk of approaching that feeling that was (up to that time) unacceptable to him.

LN: You are talking about the situations we mentioned earlier, in which the ego tends not to relate to the self.

SB: Exactly.

LN: This talk makes me think of anxiety pathologies in our time.

SB: That's right. The physical equivalent of this is the colic of a hollow organ. The hollow organs, the stomach, the intestines, the bladder, when they contract in a spasm or suffer an obstruction (a gallbladder or kidney stone, a mechanical gastrointestinal occlusion), they tense up: they tense up to such an extent that the subject feels, in addition to pain, tremendous anguish, because he feels that he cannot free himself from that tense state.

When at last the hollow organ can let out the contents that were previously stuck and not drainable, the individual provides a sense of enormous well-being and liberation. The moment our patients are able to cry—to tell the truth, this is not the only phenomenon with which this happens, but it is the most frequent, because it is directly associated with psychic sadness—and they get in touch with the feeling, they are in the presence of the affection behind it, and alone the anguish goes away. The experience, the real feeling, remains.

LN: You have translated depersonalisation as the non-pathological situations in which the ego is somewhat lost: the boundaries with the other become more blurred, but without an unpleasant sense of confusion. There are, on the other hand, other situations in which the analyst has to be there without saying so, because his or her emotional presence as "another in the room" is unacceptable, and then one struggles to make the we feel.

SB: Indeed.

LN: I think of your article "The bar in the desert" (2005), and I am reminded of adolescent patients and those with more fragile narcissism, for whom the we—that is, the recognition of being in rapport with an analyst who is emotionally other than oneself—is like kryptonite for Superman. Would you like to tell us about cases in which a discrete otherness is appropriate?

SB: You mentioned—and I thank you— "The bar in the desert", where I talk about the situations in which the analyst should not expect to fill the scene or even to be its director, but should allow himself to be used at most as an object, or as a background actor that gives value to the subject.

I remember Gian Carlo Zapparoli, an important Italian author who was also recognised abroad as an expert in the treatment of psychosis (he also had an IPA award), talking about this aspect in the early 1980s. He was sitting in a chair at the Centro Veneto di Psicoanalisi, which at that time was the home of its founder Giorgio Sacerdoti; we were all listening and he stated very resolutely, "If curing a session a severe, psychotic patient wants us to be a chair, we at that moment have to be a chair".

Translation: if the patient, clearly a severe patient, does not tolerate you being an animate, separate, autonomous being in relation to him, or even worse, that you are able to condition him, and if you want him to be there with you, and for some form of psychic coexistence to begin, you must agree to become an inanimate, inert object, at his complete disposal (precisely, like a chair …), without any ambitions of protagonism of any kind. You have to stand there and listen. Just be.

He argued that this attitude must be held—if necessary—for a long time, so that the patient, a little at a time, can familiarise himself with that cohabitation and, who knows, sooner or later, give a sign of life or recognition to the other. In saying this, however, Zapparoli is talking about decidedly serious patients.

LN: "Doctor," a hypothetical patient might say, "how can you give me today what I did not have when I needed it? And if you cannot give it to me, should I simply resign myself to never having it?"

SB: One has to see what the patient is asking for or wants. Sometimes the requests are impossible, and it will not be possible to meet them. I previously spoke about a patient who seemed to be like those pandas who can only feed on the leaves of a certain kind of bamboo. Perhaps it was I who was unable to find it, that bamboo. I also had the feeling, however, that this person really cultivated a desire, an impossible, omnipotent expectation: that she wanted to drink the sea, to inglobate everything. I still don't know what the truth was.

LN: As I was talking to a brilliant colleague, Anna Cordioli, about the conversation I was preparing to have with you, she said, "You know, find a way to discuss the fact that he gives the impression of being too good. So many analysts today seem to me to have become too 'mummy'". She added that once, at a congress, she heard you say that with a certain patient we need to go back to a pre-oral, almost amniotic stage. But if we promote regression to the origins of unmet needs, our colleague would say, don't we risk promoting narcissistic fixation to bamboo, instead of leading towards progression?

SB: Certainly the risk is there. As we have already said, the fact that analysts specialise, in a more or less unconscious and preferential way, in configuring developmental, relational, and even drive scenarios of a certain kind or level congenial to them, is a real risk.

There was a period when, to put it in somewhat of a caricature, French analysts threw it all on the primary scene, English analysts went straight to lactation or even earlier, and certain American intersubjectivist analysts, on the other hand, made fairly recurrent use of a very frank exchange between patient and analyst, understood as two already well-constituted subjects, regardless, perhaps, of what the actual evolutionary levels of the interlocutors were from moment to moment.

I am talking about cases (and there would be many others) in which it might have been recognisable that there was a certain stereotype in the scenario, in the phantasmatic relational profile that was going on, somewhat like the situation I mentioned of the sommelier who proposed the same wine to everyone.

The overall portrayal of the therapeutic scenario, on the other hand, should also and above all relate to the specific patient and the stage he or she is going through, whilst recognising that each analyst has his or her own specificity, his or her own formative history, and his or her own well-characterised theoretical–clinical toolkit.

I have come across some patients in whom the problem was, with all evidence, predominantly oedipal: these people did not lack a fundamental sense of self, nor the capacity for a two-way relationship, but rather the capacity to relate to each other and to live together if there were more than two of them. Aspects of rivalry, jealousy, exclusion, castration, or vices of triumph over rivals dominated the scene. In the more problematic cases, it could certainly have been argued whether that intense oedipal conflict might have been the consequence of an earlier preoedipal stage in which a strong internal split between "good object" and "bad object" had been formed in the child, later reproduced in a similar split between the internal parental figures, with a "good" father and a "bad" mother, or vice versa. Certainly, it is a clear and potentially interesting dynamic-evolutionary pattern, in which one could clearly read the overdetermined roots and pathogenetic pathways that had resulted in, for example, a particularly pronounced, exaggerated Oedipus that was difficult to manage in adulthood. But in some cases, however, the impression was that the earlier stages had taken place quite naturally, and that instead in the oedipal stage the growth process had been somewhat arrested, that at that moment there had been an obstacle, some fracture, a clash, an impact that could not be experienced in a natural way.

There are many situations in which we are confronted in session with the effective seductiveness of a hysterical patient, or with a strong erotic arousing transference of a neurotic quality (not an erotised transference, which would be pregenital, psychotic in quality and in fact un-seductive, if anything asphyxiating); in the erotic trans-ference, indeed, the person has achieved sufficiently genital seductive competence, but is reluctant to accept the oedipal defeat and demise. In other cases, we are grappling with a male patient who at some point on their developmental path does not accept the natural oedipal sunset period, and resolutely insists on denying the existence and function of the "third party". In both of these scenarios becoming a "mammo" certainly does not go well. There is an obstacle there to be dealt with politely and tactfully, but one of a very different nature from one who has suffered caregiving deficits.

If, on the other hand, with a traumatically shaken, poorly integrated, we can even say decompensated patient, we pretend to provide a non-maternal relational environment and care from the start, without a focus on Central Ego functioning or recovery of the state of the Self, in my opinion it is not a question of being a "mammo" or not, but of recognising what is actually needed: if it is a person who is still far behind in growth, some restraining and nurturing functions are necessary.

In short, a proper caring relationship should form and organise itself according to the specific needs of the person with whom and for whom we are working, otherwise it will end up precisely selling everyone the same wine. An analyst, therefore, should have diverse theories, internal arrangements, and technical tools.

LN: We are talking about building the possibilities for a coexistence that is tolerable, from case to case, according to the needs of each patient. I think of the concept of truth, which Bion argues is food for the mind. I ask you two questions about it: what rapport do you have with truth and with lying in psychoanalysis? How much truth can be tolerated?

SB: An expression I like to use is "enduring reality", drawn from the title of a work by Loredana Micati (1993), who in turn was inspired by a line in T. S. Eliot's poem "Burnt Norton". That phrase takes us forward in our response, because undoubtedly the concept of truth must always be understood in terms of its possible liveability and tolerability. If we were all nourished with truths that we cannot bear—and there are, for everyone, truths that we cannot bear—our minds would react God knows how, and not necessarily in a developmental way.

What rings true and right, in Bion's consideration, is that a few spoonfuls of truth, as many as are digestible by the person at that moment, are those that nourish; however, if I offer *salama da sugo*—a very spicy sausage of the Ferrara Renaissance, reserved in our days for iron stomachs—to an infant, I am not doing him a good service; it will be necessary to wait until he grows up before he can taste, appreciate, and digest such a food.

LN: In this regard I would elaborate on another dimension that you have included alongside that of interpsychic. And, therefore, I ask you, what is the relationship between too much truth, trauma, and the concept of transpsychic, which recalls a violent intrusion?

SB: The three expressions are potentially synonymous, or at least they pertain to the same dimension, which is pathological and destructive: administering too much truth can mean traumatising someone and putting something inside them that does not follow the possible and natural metabolic pathways.

For example, with Covid-19, a kind of unconscious collective test was unleashed regarding vaccine-related anxieties of alteration or poisoning. There was a part of the population, regardless of cultural, educational, or other level, that associated the idea of the prick injecting a preparation for the experience of potential danger to the integrity of the bodily self; that it could intoxicate, poison.

In this situation, the transpsychic is—in terms of psychic equivalents—that which you cannot control in the mouth, nor can you monitor with cognitive functions in its qualities and components, nor can you digest it, because it is put directly into your bloodstream. These aspects of the vaccine device produce anguish in all those who distrust, in the object relationship, the power of the object over their own self: fantasies of the object's overpowering the subject are conjured up, in the sense that the subject could not control its own somatopsychic boundaries, and fears that alien elements would be propounded, inoculated, and traumatically imposed upon it by which the other could replace the subject's own self by possessing, constraining, and determining it beyond measure.

The ultimate regressive fantasy is that of the microchip, as in certain science fiction movies; and the ultimate phantom, in my opinion, is that of total dependence on the object, which would then become the indefinite master of the subject's Self: "Grrrrrr!!! Mother, you want me to be totally dependent on you! And I don't accept that!" (this is what we would call the original polemical relation to the object).

Of course, this discourse does not detract from the fact that there may be objective aspects, more or less real, in the complete issue of vaccines; let us not enter that field now. But when fear prevails beyond normal evidence and proportions, I find myself translating this feeling even more specifically, in relational terms, with an expression like:

> Oh, Object! You would like to put things inside me in a way that is not one that I can control through the cognitive capacities of my mouth. You want to pierce a tissue of mine and, therefore, alter the integrity of my container, the skin, and directly inoculate me with this stuff. So, I should fully trust you, but in fact I distrust you: so I will never accept or employ this mode of yours.

The important thing is that this disposition of mind can consolidate, crystallise, and become an unconscious fixed pattern that repeats itself punctually and with rigid typicality in the person's life, determining his or her character and relational style.

CHAPTER 7

Questions of style

LN: Whilst I am reflecting about the difficulty of introjecting something one does not know enough, without having control over it, I think about the patient you were speaking about, who needed the analyst to be a chair, and about the necessity for a tolerable truth, otherwise, as you say, "The mind reacts God knows how". Rejection, closure, or whatever.

There are patients who have an occluded mind, unavailable to the contribution of the other, because they have no relational space available to them. In these cases, you propose to create that space that is not there, that is, to "construct the analytic patient".

SB: This is an expression first used by Fred Busch (2016). It puts the focus as much on the possibilities as on the patient's initial difficulties of working in analysis.

So, we are grappling with an expression that defines a very current concept, that of a fundamental operation of creating the conditions for developing analytic thinking. Give us two tips on the kind of work you use to expand the patient's capacity to accommodate content, symbols, emotions. A suggestion on style, small or big tricks?

In general, patients learn a great deal from hearing how the analyst experiences psychic space and how he or she does or does not make it available to them: in order for them to develop a mental container for their own emotions and thoughts, it is essential to provide them with the genuine experience of being housed in a mind that is willing to accommodate them.

If the analyst agrees to listen to the patient, without the pretence of reacting immediately and providing answers even for long periods of time, with that perceptible listening he or she begins to create the experience of an inner space, a container, a non-intrusive presence.

To realise how far from obvious this is, we need only think of what commonly happens when a person meets someone he or she knows on the street and starts talking to him or her about a difficulty they have: more often than not, the interlocutor allows him or her to express himself for a rather short time, after which he interrupts him to explain what he should do or—even more invasively—to tell him what has happened to him, quickly substituting his own self-centred subjectivity for his own, usually to silence him and to get away with more or less plausible summary and hasty formulations. That does not happen in analysis, and it is a substantial difference. But there is more. The analyst can also provide the sensation and experience of these relational aspects, widening the spaces created in the exchange, through what I have described as tools or technical expedients.

For example, when we, listening to the patient, occasionally say "mmmh", we are signalling that we are there and listening, that we savour his words and are interested in him going on with his associations. We don't set out on the spur of the moment to tell him what we have been thinking, what we think of what he is thinking; rather, we leave additional space for him to express himself (from the Latin ex-premere, that is, for him to press something out of himself that will come into us, like the espresso coffee). In this way, we implicitly give the idea that we have an internal space that welcomes, in which the patient can send in things of his own, which can then be brought into play again between the two of us.

Another example is when we ask for clarification through expressions such as "Such as? Such as? For example?" In this case we urge him to proceed with the exploratory and associative work, asking him to extend it, to persist in that direction, precisely because it is working in making us imagine or feel what he has inside.

Perceiving the analyst's inner space is the experience that helps the patient not to rush into giving us an answer right away without having first listened at least a little to himself: the patient's ego learns from the analyst's way of working to give some space to other inner parts of himself.

LN: With this brief roundup of examples, as well as with the work in recent years, it seems to me to be testifying to the fact that the therapeutic and maturational function of psychoanalysis is not so much understanding as experiencing. This idea unites the work of many contemporary analysts. Can we think that, given the self as the experiencing instance, it is the site of the greatest changes in psychoanalysis?

SB: Here, no! This would be in my opinion too narrow a formulation.

My view is that the main purpose of analysis is not only experience-making, but fostering the transformation of the relationship between the patient's Ego and Self: we must help every human being to have a broader, more fluid, more alive, and creative relationship between their Central Ego and their Self, with his experiences, his experiential sense of Self. Because the patient's Central Ego has its own extreme importance, dignity, and usefulness. Only, as long as it was the only interlocutor considered worthy of attention, the rest of the Self, the rest of the person, was not properly contacted.

Maybe we provided the Central Ego with a quantity of information, directions or interpretations that were descriptive enough, but these were not felt by the patient as sufficiently in harmony and in touch with all parts of the self.

On the other hand, if we gave space only to the self and the lived experience, we might overlook the need for the Central Ego to preside over the transitions between inside/outside, between various parts of the person, between self and others, between reality and fantasy, and the regulation of drives: that is, to adequately perform the functions that are proper to it, and that enable the subject to conduct himself and make sense of things.

That is why, in my opinion, when we talk about "working with the ego", we describe situations in the session in which we make the point on the map together with the patient's ego to say more or less where we are: to say what mountains are those there, what river is this one here, to give a recognisable meaning to the experience.

But it's also true that in analysis, when things are going sufficiently well, we don't just see things, concepts, ideas on the map: if we work with the Self, we immerse ourselves in the landscape, we walk through meadows, we go up and down mountains, we dive into the water, we also experience.

I think one of the key words in today's psychoanalysis is "integration".

LN: In a conversation we had a few years ago, Thomas Ogden told me that it rarely helps the patient to understand why he or she does anything, since this is a form of cause/effect, linear type of communication, whereas, he added, "we don't experience things, within ourselves, through linear thinking". I interpreted these statements as putting an accent on an aspect of the work that values emotional expression alongside knowledge of one's mental mechanisms.

On the other hand, following what you are saying, I sense the need to integrate the kind of work that Ogden calls ontological, with the moments in which the patient is helped to understand himself, i.e. a more epistemological moment. What are your thoughts on this?

SB: Yes. I believe that part of the enhancement of the experience of psychoanalysis that Ogden (2019) calls ontological depends on the fact that we have had an excess of knowledge in the average development of the human mind and culture. For this reason, recovering the more experiential aspects takes on a value today that is often experienced as superior; this, however, does not mean neglecting the Central Ego and the bundle of cognitive mental functions that are proper to it (precisely, the epistemological side of psychoanalysis). I think knowledge has its importance if it is integrated with experience. Of course, if it instead works against the latter, then we are not there, there is a dissociative or even oppositive level. But if the two dimensions are integrated, we have a further level of maturation and harmonisation.

Let me give you an example. When I used to travel for analysis, between Venice and Casalecchio di Reno, I would take the train. On the return trip from Bologna to Venice, I would run into companies of Japanese tourists doing the classic Rome, Florence, and Venice circuit in less than two days. These people had visited Paris, London, and Berlin in the previous three days, and they were in a state of total confusion. They were exchanging with each other models of the Colosseo, of gondolas, of the David, of the Eiffel Tower, no longer able to figure out where, what, and how. The experience from them had certainly been intense and powerful—they had been in front of monuments of enormous historical and scenic impact—but it was not at all integrated with knowing what, where, and how they were.

Once they arrived in Venice, they defended themselves from the fascinating and alienating encounter with this city so absurdly different from the rest of the world by constantly taking photographs. It was a way of not being "in" or "with" Venice, it was a paroxysmal, continuous, and botched attempt to register in a cognitive dimension, made up of images that were meant to ensure the control of experiential overexposure and indigestion through cognitively collecting those places.

There was, in many of those dazed tourists, an obvious difficulty in integrating the cognitive level with the experiential one: integrating them would have meant feeling, in that case, all the magic and strangeness of Venice, which then can be better understood by knowing its history, knowing the how and or why of its conformation, and yet at the same time feeling the smells, the voices, the special flavours of a cuisine that has been originally constructed in that environment: that is, by directly experiencing Venice, possibly with the ego and the self, but with the necessary calm …

Integration is, from this point of view, a further goal than the almost traumatic jolt of the first impact with an unknown reality so different from what one is used to.

In my opinion, many authors, including Ogden who is serving us as a reference in this case, have outlined aspects that one was previously unable to describe, imagine, represent, conceptualise, or even feel.

Each of them has added a piece, to this increasingly deepening and complex cognitive process; so much so that we do not throw away many of the Freudian notions, we simply do not consider them as the ultimate goal, but go beyond.

Melanie Klein, Winnicott, Bion, Kohut, and many others have described configurations and processes that are true and serve us.

At this point, however, "transference to individual authors" comes into play, leading to the selection, privileging, and emphasising of certain scenarios, certain concepts, certain aspects at the expense of others, based on feelings of cultural familiarity, affiliation, and belonging.

None of us can be encyclopaedic; besides, we are our parents' children, for goodness sake, we are not everyone's children.

And so, it should not surprise or shock us that every analyst has his or her favourite theoretical referents.

LN: Whoever the analysts' theoretical referents are, there are conceptions and phenomena inescapable for psychoanalysis. One of these is the dream. You edited a now landmark monograph by Boringhieri, recently republished by Mimesis. The title *The Dream One Hundred Years Later* (2016).

As with analytic conversation and analytic dialogue, can we speak of a progressive shift from the dream understood mostly as a site of analysable content to the dream as an experience of self?

SB: Indeed, yes! *The Interpretation of Dreams* is one of those great classics in which we see that what Freud said is not at all outdated, quite the contrary! It is just that these are not the only possible discoveries about dreaming.

So many authors have pointed out not only the function of the dream as wish fulfilment, or the work of the dream as a masking of these desires or drives, as Freud argued. There are other dimensions of the dream that have gradually been known, such as that of making experience, because the dream is not real, but it is true, it is experiential.

If we really dream something well, we can expect a new experience.

In an unpublished paper I have just presented at the Florence Psychoanalytic Center, "The dream as experience", I enjoyed quoting the observation made by Dement (2001) on the case of a golfer. This player, with a very advanced technique, had repeatedly tried to change a certain detail in his playing setup, without succeeding. He didn't know why he couldn't do it, but he just couldn't. We are talking about the finesse of high specifications; however, despite his conscious efforts he could not achieve the desired result. Then comes a night when the player dreams nonstop about how to execute that shot. He goes to the golf course and … the shot succeeds! Jokingly, I thought he might comment, "No wonder, I worked eight hours on it last night".

The dream was not a real event, it was not the same as being on the golf course, but it was true as an internal experience; it was true, probably, at the level of internal connections between who-knows-what circuits, and as such it allowed for authentic modification.

Also, in "The dream as experience" I cited the fact of a patient of mine who had not had sexual intercourse for more than ten years, due to a very complicated series of situations with the wife and because of certain unconscious limitations he had towards his own sensuality. In the dream he finally felt a powerful emotion, because he was able to experience a love situation with a desirable and desiring woman. The next day he was a different person because he had experienced something similar to a real love encounter. He knew he had not really experienced it, but he had really experienced it.

LN: I think of the fear that so many patients have when they experience erotic dreams with people who are not their partners.

SB: Well, of course, some are scared to death. How many insomnias are due to the vague (and actually not erroneous …) perception of the risk of dreaming about something that may be sexual, may be aggressive, may be upsetting about the imagine of self … In short, something that patients would really risk experiencing if they dreamed.

LN: Still staying in the area of eros, among your interests is reflection on the quality of transference: you wrote about loving, erotic, erotised transference (Bolognini, 1994). You later developed the theme in a second work, which is illuminating for me, in which you talk about erotisation as a consequence of impossible contact (Bolognini, 2012).
You wrote about those situations in which the erotisation of a relationship is the extreme attempt to have contact with the other, when no alternative can be found. So, recovering a dimension of warm welcome reduces the need to experience the relationship with the object in a highly erotised way.

SB: From a certain point of view, in the true erotised transference, not the erotic one, the desire is not truly sexual: it is a desire for control, for total adherence to the object and vice versa, in short, for possession. It can be similar to what certain French authors, such as Paul Denis, call *pulsion d'emprise*, which there and then seems to be a love affair, a matter between man and woman.

It is actually a matter between subject and object, where the subject is very regressed and has an archaic need to control and possess the object. So, the analyst, if he is the object of an erotised transference, feels after a while (perhaps after gassing himself narcissistically by deluding himself that he has aroused a great attraction in the patient) a great sense of weight and constraint, because he feels that in that relationship the object (the analyst) ends up being enslaved, possessed, taken captive.

Instead, in the erotic, through seduction, the subject's need to disprove the defeated oedipal, that is, that stage, physiological for everyone, which sees the dusk of the Oedipus and the entry into the latency stage, which from the age of 5, 6 years reaches puberty. That stage is not accepted by some boys and girls, who do not submit to the idea that there is a conjugal relationship between the father and mother, and who struggle all their lives, once they grow up, to deny the fact that they were not (and, in the timelessness of the unconscious, are still not be) the one preferred to that other, to the oedipal competitor.

In those cases, the triadic pattern in which the subject must ensure that he or she has a superior seductive power, which will defeat the opponent and confirm him or her in his or her victorious narcissism, is different from that of the erotised transference in one crucial specific respect: usually, the person who develops an erotised transference is an individual who has had a very poor relational treatment, so he needs to start over from the beginning by possessing the object in a primary fusion appropriate to his needs that he could not experience in due time.

In contrast, those who develop erotic transference have acquired seductive competence because they have been loved by the parent of the opposite sex, and they do not want to lose that privilege and illusion of total oedipal victory.

The latter must always compulsively confirm to himself that he has a *passe-partout*, a valid passport to all states; and he is, in any case, a person with valid attractiveness. He is not an unhappy person, narcissistically ill-equipped and doomed to defeat, like the erotised person: in fact, he is seductive to the analyst. In this case, the analyst does not feel any oppression, rather he develops fantasies (we would be the most beautiful couple in the world, we could run away together, etc.). Since, in addition to the analyst's own transference, if any, there is a transference contribution from the patient, the patient is able to induce this loving experience in the therapist, especially when the latter suffers from narcissistic vulnerabilities that are little analysed, or reactivated by events in his life.

LN: One of the most important changes over these recent decades concerns a kind of axiom of our method, namely that in analysis one does not act, but speaks. Here, this sort of taboo of yesteryear—assuming it was such, because we know that analysts of the past acted more than they were given credit for—is becoming very blurred. Back then, it was argued that the patient, on the couch, should inhibit motor discharge (thus movements, actions, gestures) as much as possible, in favour of verbal expression. You write that "today we do not denounce so much the motor discharge, but we understand the equivalent of action". Do we talk about that?

SB: Yes. Whilst the more fundamentalist circles, especially in a radical part of French psychoanalysis, had come to say that any movement, even of the little toe, was a yielding to motor discharge, subsequently the issue has been challenged by the growing conception that we actually do something all the time, not in a muscular sense but in a relational sense. After all, it was in France that Racamier (1988) explored the concept of "talking action".

Jay Greenberg, one of the leading North American exponents of relational psychoanalysis, has been arguing for fifteen years already that the analyst is always doing something: for example, he talks or does not speak, speaks a lot or speaks little, uses one tone of voice or uses another. Through words he communicates the equivalent of actions, but he does it anyway.

This is not to dismiss the coarse actions, the acting out*, that impulsively substitute for thought, but rather to understand the equivalences between elements that are not actions in the motor sense, but are in the relational sense. If I talk to the patient in one way or another, I do something: there is not just a theoretical, abstract utterance.

LN: Your assertion that the analyst "does it anyway" prompts a question for me about the concept of neutrality*. I am not so much talking about abstinence* as I am talking about neutrality understood as the equidistance of the analyst from the different internal parts of the patient. I wonder, and I ask you, how much neutrality is still a cornerstone of psychoanalytic intervention and how differently it is defined than it was long ago.

SB: The claim to be completely neutral is utopian and unrealistic, in fact, but it retains its profound inspirational ideal function.

In a sense, the concept of neutrality has been enriched with more complex technical declinations. For example, the enhancement of the ability to suspend, waiting for what will become apparent shortly thereafter, instead of rushing hastily into the material that emerges in session when one is not yet able to understand and work with it, remains a fundamental point of analytic technique. Maintaining a certain equidistance on the part of the analyst towards the characters in a scene narrated by the patient, without taking early sides in favour of one or the other protagonist in the conflict, whilst resonating emotionally in a natural way, is also a setup in the service of the ideal of neutrality.

The analyst differs from any interlocutor, in session, precisely by virtue of his or her equidistributional availability in his or her contact with the various parts of the patient's Self, a suspension, even in listening, of what comes from his or her internal objects or egosyntonic* Defensive Ego.

For example, it is quite common for the patient to present us with a split scenario in which the object is all bad and the patient's conscious ego is all good.

If we ally ourselves in a "goodist" way only with the patient's conscious ego (aka ego-syntonic concordant setup), we lose a good chunk of him, a chunk that has usually been projected onto the object.

If we conversely distrust the patient's Central Ego too systematically (the so-called "psychoanalysis of suspicion"), then we lose touch with that part of him.

Suspension helps us to understand it better, to see what develops along the way.

In this sense, the analyst tends to value and develop a capacity for suspension, and for continuous exploration, which is not satisfied with what appears at first glance.

At the countertransferential level, we can resonate in a concordant or complementary way, or both, and then it is even better, because we can get a more in-depth view of the complexity of the various components in the field.

When our general practitioner visits us, he needs, during palpation or as he reads the results of the laboratory tests, to maintain some suspension before reassuring us or alarming us with a response: if he is a good doctor, he needs to explore the various aspects of the situation as best he can, he needs to feel whether the abdomen is treatable, what the liver is like, he needs to feel whether it hurts there, or not.

If he were to reassure us right away, he would certainly not be the best doctor. This is a very trivial example, however, the analyst can collect an inspirational model of this kind as well: that of a physician who is capable of not taking a premature departure by shooting off guesses in the dark, and of not predicting a serious diagnostic hypothesis until the picture has become clear in all its components.

Which is by no means to be cold, because the ways in which an examination is conducted by a physician can also vary infinitely. We may be faced with a chilling doctor who from beginning to end does not move a muscle in his face or utter a word; or a more humane doctor, who does not get out of line until he has made up his mind about the situation, but whom we feel is communally at work with us and on us.

Cooperation, and even the concept (much criticised by some) of therapeutic alliance*, serve neutrality. The alliance, after all, does not consist of always agreeing with the patient by agreeing with his conscious state and confirming his already defensively consolidated way of seeing things; rather, it consists of agreeing to explore together: which is quite another thing.

LN: Why do you say that the therapeutic alliance is a concept that has been so criticised by some?

SB: Because some felt that it favoured an imbalance in the analyst's capacity for abstinence as opposed to the desired neutrality. I cite an incident from many years ago.

An aspiring colleague, who had been in analysis with me for some years, went for selection interviews to enter training. He rang the door of an analyst from another city, whom he did not know, to undergo one of the three interviews by which he would be judged suitable or not. When the door was opened for him, the young aspirant (now an experienced colleague) held out his hand to exchange a civil good morning, as he was accustomed to do with me when I welcomed him to the office. The other pretended not to notice and held his hands firmly beside his body.

It would have been different if there had been a "freeze" from both sides; instead, in this case one of the two (the weaker one, at that moment) had exposed himself for a conventional greeting, and in my opinion, to remain still was a fairly strong action, if not an actual act. At this point, the young aspirant, already somewhat embarrassed, said: "Good morning, I am such-and-such". And the other, without moving a muscle in his face, replied, "It's obvious". As if to say: if you show up at this hour, then it is obvious that you are that person. Yes, agreed it is obvious, however, it is also true that if you answer in that way you are also definitely unpleasant, you are not neutral.

"You're doing something", Greenberg would perhaps say. You're doing something repulsive, chilling.

You can conduct a selection interview with respect, with restraint, and with neutrality, without it meaning bias, without forgetting that both of us are people, me and him. Maybe I won't dwell on it, but humanly I will accept it with a "Good morning, have a seat". Instead, that recruiter, in my opinion, really thought he was behaving in a "perfectly neutral" way.

LN: Without forgetting the concept of metasetting*, which is that we live in a world with rules, customs that we all perceive as normal.

SB: Exactly, yes. Which doesn't mean making it easy: "Look, come here, I've already figured out that you're fine the way you are". No. We are here to explore, to understand, to bring out, to make sense, to do in short a complex work … But between people.

CHAPTER 8

Psychoanalytic training

LN: We have sketched some epochal changes, over a century that has exponentially altered the external reality and also the internal realities of people. Changes not only social, but also psychoanalytic changes, in the way of posing of patients, of the way of approaching the analytic process. Do you think that the training of analysts should adapt to the changes we have talked about by presenting something new, or do you think that our training is already suitable and that the attention that analysts learn to have respect for the new things that emerge in the course of the analytic process is enough?

SB: I have noticed big differences between different psychoanalytic societies and schools.

The SPI, for example, offers such a variety of models, of approaches, of styles, of ways of being among its analysts that it is difficult for a candidate not to come into contact during training with all these different modalities.

During seminars he or she may feel and experience a structuring Freudian methodological rigour, or he or she may encounter a Bionian type of creativity; he or she may come in contact with the dimension of the intermediate territory between patient and analyst, of exchange, in the Winnicottian type of play, as an additional way of working.

Or again: the student may experience the perceptible attention of the Kohutian analyst to the narcissistic state of the self, whereby patients with a grandiose* self will be expected until this is deflated. I am citing models that may concern different authors, as you can well imagine.

LN: The SPI, of which we are a part, has developed by importing analytic modes and cultures from different countries, so our psychoanalysis does not have a pedigree, in fact, it is very composite.

Instead, there are societies that have established distinct and recognisable autonomous schools, such as the French society or the English society.

How do you think we can hold together under one umbrella, the one represented by the IPA and which we can more generally call Freudian or post-Freudian psychoanalysis, the plurality of theoretical models that have developed over the course of the last century? Some would like more uniform training models and more rigid paths. Others would prefer to value the languages and analytic dialects of individual countries: we have a tradition of medieval communes, the French had the Empire, and so on.

You, who were first on the board (which is a kind of parliament) and then president of the IPA, have always shown an interest in these issues.

SB: I cannot help but go back in my memory to all the experiences I have had over the years, and I will describe them shortly, to give an idea of the realities I have encountered and on which I will express some opinions.

When it was possible to travel without particular difficulty—and thus before Covid-19—those who had an institutional function, as I had as president of the IPA, sooner or later visited almost every society in the world; and the visit followed its own fairly standard programme, which included, after arrival, a dinner with the society's elders. That was a very interesting first intake, a taste of the local societal atmosphere.

The next day, in the morning, there was the official, institutional, administrative part, with the Executive of the Society; whilst in the afternoon the scientific meetings began with the presentation of theoretical and clinical work, and then with the discussion of clinical cases in a seminary situation. That was the time when the climate, style, history, and language of each analytic family, national or local, effectively emerged.

For me this exploratory experience was of enormous interest, so much so that in the last year of my presidency I spent almost a month in Latin America, visiting the various societies and their locations. Before that

I had done something similar by invitation in North America, as well as naturally in Europe.

I would summarise the result as follows: I realised the fact that there are excellent analysts in every country, and that the level of reliability, competence, and even analytical culture is now high everywhere.

This is the result of many factors: for example, the fact that in recent times scientific papers have been translated into many languages and disseminated widely, thanks to the IPA network, even in remote areas. Moreover, before the restrictions due to Covid-19, invitations to the most representative analysts of the various societies had been very frequent.

Much credit for this had been the CAPSA (an acronym for the Committee of Analytic Practice & Scientific Activities), the IPA initiative to fund intercontinental exchanges between different societies, allowing northern and South American analysts to meet with European societies, working together with local colleagues; and conversely making it possible for Europeans to go overseas, on a rotating basis, for a virtuous process of mutual scientific cross-fertilisation. This was a great initiative that greatly deprovincialised the environment of many local analytical communities.

To this, we must then add a second proactive factor, namely, the increasingly widespread knowledge of foreign languages. Today there are a great many analysts (especially young ones) who speak and understand English sufficiently, but also Spanish, which has become the second intercontinental IPA language, and a little French as well.

Thus was realised the opportunity not only to read foreign papers, but also to hear analysts trained in other educational settings speak live, to discuss with them, and to fully perceive the climates and mentalities of other analytic families. This constituted a momentous opportunity for enrichment for all of us.

Like others before me, I was able to see for myself that, if one works on the clinical material, today's discussion is much more interactive and less dogmatic than it used to be, and it no longer runs aground on theoretical issues that tended to become rather often "theological", real religious wars.

In the past, the way one often worked for the other "was not psychoanalysis". Today, it is much rarer to hear this accusation resounded in official venues, except in a few pockets of fundamentalism, because it has been recognised that the elements of general knowledge of psychoanalysis, common to analysts all over the world, are many more than the points of difference.

On the clinical material, then, the understanding is usually the result of interesting and reasoned interchange in the discussion groups, which very often arrive—after long work—at something consensual, albeit with natural "distinctions". The biggest problems arise, on the other hand, when one enters too frontally and head-on, into the area of authorial devotions or totemic phallicities. Let me explain. Just as for children one's daddy and mommy are untouchable, so for the most regressive part of all analysts are one's trainers, reference authors, and idealised maestros sacred and untouchable, and hold the truth. It is that process by which once (no longer today) elementary school children used to say, "… but the teacher said that!" To say that what was stated had to be true, without any doubt whatsoever.

There is less of a disposition to sacrality among analysts today, which perniciously resurfaces, however, when one speaks in theoretical terms only: then dogmatic "fouls" rise again and confront each other in the open field, with threats of mutual castration.

If, on the other hand, one speaks more in clinical terms, then after some time of exploratory discussion one realises that an inevitable and unexpected mix of potentially useful concepts has been realised, such that the terms of the question under consideration are reformulated as much as the participants' own starting scientific/identiary profiles.

Over the past two decades, there has been a fading of an inveterate cliché: once, for example, it was classic for Americans to think that the French were only philosophers, and in turn for the French to think that North Americans were yes-or-no psychotherapists. As for South Americans, they were so little known (apart from José Bleger and a few others) that they created no problems, in the sense that they hardly existed in the minds of their colleagues on other continents. Today, fortunately, this is no longer the case.

The summation of these changes results in the fact that when the analyst returns to work with his patients after these clinical interchanges, he is no longer exactly equal to when he left, days before, for that conference.

LN: I was accompanied throughout your narrative by a free association. When you said: "There are very good analysts everywhere", the expression one often hears in football rang in my head: in the international arena there are no longer "mattress teams", those against whom anyone wins effortlessly.

SB: Yes, that's exactly right!

LN: Let's stay in football. You know when you hear the various coaches like Cruyff, or Sacchi, or the other devotees of the beautiful game talking, and maybe in the end you end up getting beaten by a weaker team that plays "*al catenaccio*", that is, defensively, typically Italian and much maligned?

Well, this fantasy answered for itself the question I was going to ask you. I was going to ask a dry question: one psychoanalysis or more psychoanalysis? Then I thought that Brazilian football is very different from English football, and critics can spend hours dissecting the differences in approach and traditions, but in the end the basic rules are the same for all, and the team who scores more goals wins. In our case, do you win when you make the patient feel better?

SB: That's for sure.

The central point is to understand the factors of healing, the factors of cure and sanity (on which there seems to me to be some agreement in principle); these are the ones on the basis of which we can compare.

Because scientific experimental research and psychoanalysis have not always gotten along so well, the principle of authority, as you said, the *ipse dixit*, has developed, so we need to confront the clinical data to check the usefulness, precision, and clarity of conceptual apparatuses.

The scenario of theoretical debate in psychoanalysis has also changed a lot.

Just think that a concept like projective identification up to some thirty years ago could still be rejected outside the English world; in the same period, I even heard analysts say that projective identification was an abstraction with no real substrate.

Today this is no longer the case: ten years ago, when for the IPA's *Inter-Regional Encyclopedic Dictionary of Psychoanalysis* we decided to draw up an order of precedence in the presentation of the different concepts, we asked the initial seventy very qualified contributors (today there are 120) to write down in order of importance the ten notions with which they would consider it advisable to begin publication. When we compiled the rankings on the basis of that survey, projective identification was fairly far ahead; certainly not as far ahead as the unconscious or transference, but it turned out to be a concept that was also considered fundamental.

Thirty years ago, precisely, this was not the case: what was proposed by new masters of thought was confronted with the Freudian basis alone and often discarded if it did not fit the canon. Today there is more interest in a broadening of the conceptual field and theoretical and technical tools, because the cultural climate has changed.

As evidence of this, I gladly mention the fact that for as long as IPA congresses have been held, a European, a North American, and a South American were invited for plenary sessions. Well: they would each "sing their song" in the time allotted for their performance, after which they would almost close their ears to what the other two would say. Today, the panellists at the table dialogue a lot with each other, even though they come from different continents (and thus from different cultural and theoretical worlds).

The collective attitude has changed profoundly, there is a greater awareness and tolerance of what we were talking about earlier: otherness. Which used to be more difficult to accept.

LN: Before proceeding down this path, I make an aside, because you mentioned the IPA's *Inter-Regional Encyclopedic Dictionary*; which you designed and helped create.

It is a veritable reasoned dictionary, online on the IPA website, of the most important concepts in psychoanalysis. The *Dictionary* has the unique distinction of highlighting contributions from all the world's major analytic traditions.

Among other things, with a large group of colleagues we have translated several entries into Italian, which now find space on the SPI website.

I would like at this point to understand what it meant to you to devise a psychoanalytic encyclopaedia edited by the IPA, which was one of the successes of your presidency.

SB: Yes, wanting to create or at least evolve at the mondial level a truly scientific IPA based on community, not just an administrative one, was the impetus that inspired all my action in those years; and the *Encyclopedic Dictionary* was both its symbol and its product.

In fact, most of the scientific activities in the psychoanalytic field were being carried out by the national societies and continental federations, namely the EPF European, the North American APSA, and the South American FEPAL.[5]

The IPA organised its Congress every two years, but it did not perform a sufficient integrating and connecting function, in my opinion, to reduce the isolation or, if you will, even a certain theoretical narcissism of individual national communities.

The idea of making analysts and the international community aware of what all the various schools and families have produced regarding certain very important psychoanalytic concepts was a crucial goal for me.

Little was known in Europe about what was actually being done in analytic studies in Latin America or North America, and the same was true for each of the other three regions that make up the IPA (in recent years the Asia and Ocean-Pacific area has also been added, with scientific and cultural contributions of enormous interest).

Through the *Dictionary*, I wanted us to become aware of how many and what new contributions had been researched and written on these common themes.

And it is working, because analysts from various geographical areas, to our mutual surprise, now understand how much has been discovered and created in other areas of the world. Previously, it was a rather "short-lived" psychoanalysis, that is, limited to one's own backyard.

LN: It is no secret that for some time now, within the IPA, there has been an antagonism, sometimes more dialoguing, sometimes more rupturing, between different visions of psychoanalysis: more conservative, more intransigent, on the one hand, and more progressive and integrative, on the other.

I am not asking you what your position is, which seems to me to be shown by your words; rather, I am interested in the method that for you is appropriate for the dialectic to be fruitful and not divisive. We have already talked about the clinic and working together, so I would ask you to give us

---

[5] Respectively, European Psychoanalysis Federation, American Psycho-analytic Association, and Federación Psicoanalítica de América Latina.

some more details about how we can understand each other even when speaking different dialects, different languages.

SB: The focus is on working with, on, and for the object of our interest, which is a clinical object, usually a patient, a story, or a treatment.

When one begins to think in terms of the clinical object and enters into a working relationship, the narcissistic fixation rigidly restricted to one's identity-theoretical heritage of origin fades away, or at least is amortised. A greater willingness to listen to what other colleagues have to say is taking over, and this is the real royal road to knowledge and progress within an analytic community.

What profile do I have? It always comes back there: everyone has his or her own personal story, and this always inspires, at least in part, subsequent developments. I will not dwell on my childhood history: as I have also written in previous work, it is based on an extended family, with many presences of grandparents, uncles, siblings, and cousins of whom I know that I have subjectively found many later equivalents in the community environment of our international association in which I have felt—to use a rural expression—like a mouse in cheese.

I must say that I still consider myself an active part of the IPA even though I no longer have specific functions, since in the summer of 2021 I also resigned, after many years of work, from the presidency of the *Dictionary*.

This was my decision, because it is only right that others should move on, that there should be a generational change, and especially that institutional initiatives should be energised and reinvigorated by "fresh forces"; instead, I will still maintain an advisory function for some time, as is classically done in such cases to ensure some continuity with the new leaders.

I feel like an IPA analyst because I have breathed in some good in many parts of the psychoanalytic world. One might communicate, "This is a Harlequin position, which indicates so many patches of so many colours", and I reply no, it is not exactly so.

There is a substantial difference between a disarticulated and approximate eclecticism and a complex analytic culture that is aware not only of the variety of theories, but also of their less obvious functions and connections, which may combine or alternate depending on different clinical frameworks. Put in simpler words: with certain patients I am naturally reminded of certain authors, certain schools, certain experiences made in seminars, in certain places, with certain kinds of colleagues. With other patients I come up with different ones, because certain tools fit some cases very well and less well with others, and vice versa. The real problem is how ideas can be revisited, composed, and integrated within ourselves, so that there is sufficient harmony between these various parts of our personal analytical laboratory.

I mentioned to you earlier, as a last resort of the analyst in difficulty, retreating to the first topical as a very useful posture, merely observing the processes of re-emergence of contents from the unconscious and then the preconscious, awaiting developments.

There are indeed more favourable and practicable situations in which the creativity of the interpersonal relationship seems to me to be the most useful path; others in which working with shared fantasies is equally possible, at certain chosen moments. But when persecution is strong (and I feel that one cannot work with a pretence of creativity until the dust settles) then one must resign oneself to the fact that basic, noncreative containment functions are the most useful in order not to fuel persecutory tensions: at those junctures one must lower the intensity of the fire under the pot and wait for better times.

At still other times, assessing the patient's healthy or pathological narcissistic gradients, I may find another kind of theoretical support useful.

I am this way today, because I have provided these different ideas in my own analysis, heard them described very clearly and effectively in the international arena by colleagues of absolute value, recognised a usefulness, a validity, let's say even a truth in the clinic; and found my way to combine them according to a specific (psycho)analytic logic, which sometimes has not much to do—I want to say it clearly—with an Aristotelian philosophical logic.

LN: This I whisper to you: it is very difficult to be an analyst today … I can no longer say I am a young analyst, because I have just been appointed as an ordinary member [full member, a level higher than associate member, author's note], so I am no longer credible as a young person, but I still do not feel very stable. I often feel the ground crumbling under my feet, perhaps because, unlike other colleagues, I do not have a strong model to refer to. I have many friends who are excellent connoisseurs of field theory, some are refined Freudians, comfortable with their model, and sometimes I feel that it is easier for them and that they know more where to put their hands. Then I reassure myself by thinking that each of them will have their own insecurities.

I felt much relief when Antonino Ferro, our esteemed colleague with whom I had a published conversation a few years ago, told me that we could travel light and let go of so many theoretical burdens. I was fascinated by this idea, although I know that he learned theory very well so that he could then put it aside. I think that many analysts today, in such a big world with such a multiplicity of theories and approaches, find themselves displaced. Some colleagues who come to me in supervision lament how difficult it is to put together a style of work by taking a little bit from here, a little bit from there. Some envy fellow students who have become cognitivist therapists because they have stable and therefore reassuring protocols. There is a such a feeling of loss, that one feels like clinging to a rock and holding on.

SB: This is true because yours, Dr Nicoli, is an analytic generation, perhaps even a bit flooded, overwhelmed by a preponderant supply of ideas, of models, of schemes, of theories, which once were not there; new things came with the dropper, made a stir, and were more noticeable.

When I began my training, for example, discovering Klein's books was already a big event: back in Venice her theory was still little known, it was Salomon Resnik (who was shuttling between Paris and Venice after his London years) who introduced us to her.

Everyone has his or her own story, and I have the impression that your generation is perhaps in danger of being faced with an endless, huge buffet, with too many things that are also good, but impossible to taste them all.

This complicates the problem of integration, of composing one's own sufficiently harmonious line of theoretical organisation.

Cesare Musatti, one of the founders of our SPI, cited the example of plankton: he said that analysts wander here and there like cetaceans in the cultural ocean, among the various seminars, articles, texts, and so on, ending up fishing, hopefully, for something to speak to them at that moment and be of some interest and usefulness.

I think that very often that is just the way things are. After all, one can hardly expect to taste everything: everyone will have his own trajectory, his own path, his own analytical story.

LN: In this regard, I am reminded of something that you, as well as others, have mentioned. There are authors that one would never stop reading. I have three: Bolognini, Ferro, and Ogden. In you I find so much humanity, simplicity even in complexity, the clinic that I seem to practice every day. Ogden cares for every word he writes like a poet, and the same sensitivity he offers in the examples of analytical work he presents to the reader. Ferro and his "field theory" propose a very valuable freedom and creativity, which sometimes allows us to lighten the emotional burden associated with our practice.

The more I study and delve into these and other authors, the more I realise the distance between the official theories, which we learn and profess, and the unconscious ones, which we use without perhaps even realising it.

In other professions, more disciplined by strict protocols, such a reflection would be of little consequence, but in our case, given the absence of standard operating schemes or techniques, the question is particularly significant.

SB: This is a fascinating topic.

Every analyst's formative history begins with the original maternal equivalent, who is one's own personal analyst: who certainly may play now maternal, now paternal, roles and functions during analysis, but who provides a very strong primary imprinting.

Equally, the supervisors, usually equivalents of the "third", help to characterise the training experience in an incisive way.

Then come the encounters with other masters whom I have admired at seminars and conferences.

Egon Molinari, an analyst from Trieste of Hungarian origin, was my analyst; Giorgio Sacerdoti in Venice and Glauco Carloni in Bologna were my supervisors.

Later, I admired a lot of other masters of the previous generation; I could name a dozen who impressed me. Among those I met in person, I have already named Salomon Resnik, with whom I did two years of group as a patient before specialising, and whose formidable interpretative creativity struck me; then authors of great value whom I had the pleasure of meeting many times, such as Fred Busch, Ted Jacobs, Warren Poland.

I greatly admired some figures from Latin America, such as León Grinberg, Horacio Etchegoyen, Marcelo Vinhar, and my unparalleled institutional mentor Cláudio Eizirik.

Among the French, besides André Green, I owe much to Daniel Widlöcher and Haydée Faimberg.

The authors I mentioned are part of an earlier generation than mine and entered boxes of the inner world that I would call the "parental area": my transference towards them had that quality.

In the category of "siblings" many Italian and foreign colleagues have placed themselves in my internal, and the list would inevitably be boring; but what I would like to point out is the intertwining of relationships and scientific enrichment, the link between affection and knowledge inherent in our profession.

Personal relationships with some of these figures opened introjective doors that made me familiar with the concepts they proposed or ways they used them.

Just as happened in the experience of most of us with our mother, father, and significant relatives, we can recognise in this institutional transference a physiological regressive component that should not frighten us, because it has to do with some fundamental formative processes of our professional selves.

Our analytic community is truly brimming with extraordinary talents and intellectual and human resources.

And in the end the task for each of us is to be ourselves, taking into account all these paths and encounters. Then, beyond personal encounters, the magnum sea of reading opens up: that, too, can open many doors for us, especially if we are able to indulge in full immersions in the inner world that real authors know how to transmit to us and make us share; I think that in the end each of us has our own formative history, our own analytic family, our own background cultural constellation.

You certainly have it too, Dr Nicoli, don't you?

LN: I am thinking about this talk of yours about reference figures, and the world today, so confused, vast, full of contradictory information and visions. With the loss of authority of parental equivalents (institutions, teachers, stable models of reference), people are in danger of finding themselves in chaos. This applies not only to analytic training, but to the multiplication of viewpoints in every field, in mass media, on social media. So, I have noticed how transference, understood as primitive emotional reactions, is depopulating. In this complete and chaotic, there are real totems to worship. Since we are in the age of vaccines, I think of the devotees of the television virologists, and of the idols of the anti-vaxers, that Montagnier who once won the Nobel Prize ...

SB: ... and who has also spoken a lot of rubbish recently.

LN: Exactly. The world lacks the "supervisor" function to help filter, to discuss, to do critical work and synthesis. That role generally used to be played by the family doctor, the favourite teacher, a good pastor or trade unionist, a smart uncle, in short, social staples. Today, I seem to observe a tendency towards continuous salvific transference—like falling in love.

SB: True: you point out to me that, beyond the physiological transferential aspects that make one grow, there is also the opposite risk of the idealisations of the moment, desperately clinging and confusion.

LN: And later devaluations ...

SB: And devaluations. Yes, when excessive idealisations melt away like snow in the sun ...

LN: So, I too cling to his experience. With respect to your training, profession, and career as an analyst, is there anything you would not do again?

SB: This is a very difficult question, really. What would I not do again?
    Like many other Italian colleagues in the 1970s, I took an analytic path (in a concrete sense) that is difficult to imagine today, at least for those who have their analyst in the same city.
    I lived in Mestre, worked in the psychiatric hospital on the island of San Clemente in the Venice lagoon. Then I would run (so to speak, it was all a *vaporetto* ride ...) to the Santa Lucia train station and take the train. I came to Bologna station after a two-hour ride, and from there by cab to Casalecchio di Reno, where Dr Molinari resided. After the session, again cab, train, and then, for four years, a second train to Milan on

Wednesday evenings, because the training seminars were there. So, I would do a Venice–Bologna–Milan triangulation, and in the night from Milan I would take the train to Mestre.

The trip to Bologna I used to make four times a week; from a certain point of view it was a crazy life, I was always on the train, and I knew all the train controllers and commuter workers who commuted daily from one city to another. Besides, I had no choice if I wanted to become a professional, because the only other didactic analyst in the Veneto was my hospital director, Professor Sacerdoti, so I couldn't do analysis with him.

Yet, that Cyclopean effort did not seem so at the time. It is true that I was very young, but looking back on it now I wonder how I did it. There was in me an enormous force of attraction towards analysis, and not only in a narcissistic sense (in those years Italian analysts were very few), there was really a deep need, and I found in that treatment, with my analyst, what I needed.

So, for many years I lived this life. Would I do it again? Yes, if I go back in my memory to then, I would definitely do it again.

Here, if anything, I can say that certain seminars in Milan, with late-night returns, were quite a burden, because not all of them were so interesting; however, they had to be followed and so it was.

The two supervisions for me were a beautiful experience: I enjoyed them. To reach Professor Sacerdoti in Venice I used to take the bus route from the mainland plus *vaporetto* from Piazzale Roma to the island of Giudecca, and I saw Professor Carloni in Bologna on a day in which I also had the session with Dr Molinari. They were very enriching experiences. Yes, I would do it all again; they were years of evolution that were indispensable.

After that, what is it that I would not have done?

I would say nothing, the experiences of the following years (national and international seminars, congresses, study groups) I did with pleasure and conviction, in the excellent company of equally passionate and curious "brothers" and "cousins". Perhaps mine may appear to be too one-directional a description, however, I do not feel like saying, What the hell was I thinking of doing? No, because I feel that that was my path, I needed it, it was the natural development.

Even about the professional choices between psychiatry and psycho-analysis, between public and private, I have no particular regrets. At the beginning of my career, I worked in psychiatry in the psychiatric hospital in San Clemente, in the lagoon; then at the Provincial Psychotherapeutic Center in Palazzo Boldù, in Rialto, and finally as an assistant doctor in the Psychiatric Services in Treviso: all very formative experiences in contact with serious pathologies, with colleagues of considerable competence. But at some point the choice was inevitable on the organisational level, and very easy as a decision: the time had come to change jobs.

Returning to Bologna for analysis, then, was like coming home.

I am Bolognese by family and birth, and coming to do my analysis in Bologna corresponded to the recovery of a childhood experience and intergenerational heritage; and years later I moved to live here, with a sense of further reintegration.

Nonetheless, I still deeply love the Veneto region, which hosted and raised me for thirty years, where I studied from elementary school to my specialisation in psychiatry, whose dialect I speak quite well, and where I gladly return to whenever I can. To the point that I recognise myself quite well in the concluding remark of Marco Polo who, having returned to Venice after so many years of living in China, said that he felt like a Venetian in China, and eventually felt like a Chinese in Venice.

My answer, Dr Nicoli, is perhaps a bit disappointing because an interlocutor might expect something more complex or more enigmatic in reconsidering the stages of one's education But this is who I am, and this has been my formation story.

CHAPTER 9

Offline and online

LN: Your answer prompts me to ask you a question of the kind I would not have wanted to ask. It is not provocative, but it certainly asks psychoanalytic institutions to account for the current relationship between training sacrifices and professional resources. It gave me the feeling that a certain pioneering era, characterised by travels through Italy, reinforced, in those who made it through to completion, the idea isation of an object called psychoanalysis, which then became falling in love, passion. It was a time when people were not "flooded" as they are today, there was easier access to work and a greater possibility of growth.

Following the pandemic drama, as an ana ytic community we found ourselves, overnight, operating online. Sessions with patients, supervision, and conferences translated on the Web, where they partly remain to this day.

Hearing you speak of your educational labours, thinking back to my own, between Modena, Bologna, Ferrara, and Padua, I cannot help but ask if the educational future of our profession, as of so many others, will not be aided by telecommunication.

A dear colleague, also an ordinary member of the SPI, told me that he met a young man oriented towards analytic trair ing, but he lives in another city where there are no analysts. Couldn't he do online analytics? That one, maybe not, many would object, but are we sure t at for the two compulsory supervisions, of two years each, the concrete co-presences of bodies are so imperative? I gave up a supervision that I cared about, for geographical reasons. Recently, however, outside the constraints of formal training, I worked for three years with an excellent analyst in Rome, to whom I am very grateful. It would have been unthinkable for me to do this in person.

I think of how many opportunities would open up with this kind of zeroing of geographic distances, the mingling, the contamination. Letting pupils go and eat plankton from another part of the ocean, and more "tropical fish" coming to us. *Cum grano salis*, let me be clear, however, let me dream.

SB: So, I take the wide curve and start from the past. I started training analysis in 1976, and seminars and supervision in 1980. Yes, there were difficulties, such as not having a training analyst in the area, but there were also objective advantages compared to today: for example, those who worked as I did in institutions could count on considerable flexibility. Those who then had a psychoanalyst as head of service, such as Professor Sacerdoti, could distribute their working hours quite at will; thus, between night and holiday guards, morning service, and afternoon service, we could decide our own hours, as long as we respected the total number of hours. Today this is no longer the case: psychiatrists and psychologists employed in public institutions are bound to a very structured work organisation decided by others, so it would be impossible for them to go that far four times a week. They would not be able to do it.

I would add that, at the time, salaries in public service, at a rough guess, were equivalent to those of today, but at the private level what was left in the pocket of the young psychotherapeutic professional was a bit more: there was a lower tax burden and trains, petrol, and highways had lower costs, moreover with fewer queuing or parking problems when people chose the car.

The other key aspect was that high-frequency analytic patients were very easy to find. As there were few experienced specialists in the field, there was a high demand and—here I relate to what we have been talking about so far—a greater willingness of people to rely on the treatment and the analyst.

Like many young colleagues, I had also started practising psycho-therapy to pay for my own analysis, but from a certain point in the training onward I was allowed to have patients in analysis, and I remember well that they came in droves even though I was young and they did not make any resistance to adhere to the setting and the contract that was proposed to them. Today, finding a patient for three-or-four-times-a-week sessions is serious business; at that time, on the other hand, it was very easy, for colleagues who at that time were in training.

Having said that, and thus taking away some of the heroic polish from the general conditions necessary to do training back then, when there was—you are right, doctor—the narcissistic halo of pioneering, it must be acknowledged, however, that we young people back then were not pioneers at all. The analysts of previous generations, who had paved the way for the first developments of psychoanalysis in Italy, had been. On the other hand, we felt like vanguards, that is.

The issue of distance learning, however, deserves a more comprehensive discussion.

This is an issue that has always been debated within the IPA, a natural observatory since it has continuously monitored the reality of all those nations in which didactic analysts or otherwise experts were not available locally.

I am referring, for example, to all of Eastern Europe, which for many years made it necessary for therapists and psychiatrists who wanted to train themselves to face the famous shuttle analyses and travel periodically, by plane, to the European capitals where the big analytic institutes were.

Fortunately, these long training odysseys were somewhat mitigated, from a certain point on, thanks to Skype or telephone connections alternating with periods of in-person sessions.

Few may be aware that shuttle analysis had also initially had a not insignificant cost in terms of family breakups or even human lives. Some analysts from the East had died, presumably from the excessive burden of these long and frequent trips to Amsterdam, Berlin, London, and Paris, which then alternated with crazy rhythms on the days when they returned home and had to catch up on missed work. Such a lifestyle for many of them proved untenable.

The IPA board, urged by several parties, promulgated a set of new directions that later became rules even for the so-called ING (International New Groups), which is the part of the IPA that regulates training arrangements for remote countries. The council changed the previous, very restrictive regulations, which would have implied *de facto* departure from home countries for aspiring analysts, by stipulating that where there were no analysts with training functions it would be possible to design partially online training, recognised by the IPA.

Training candidates, however, had to do at least one continuous year of normal in-person analysis; after that, they could return to their country and return each year for a month or two of in-person analysis, and the rest remotely.

This change, dictated by the plan to extend psychoanalysis to distant countries, raised strong protests from the more conservative societies, which wrinkled their noses, but eventually, obtusely, signed the agreement.

The issue was not simple, however, because whilst everyone agreed that those living in more remote places in the world, especially in Asia, could not face frequent travel to go for three or four sessions a week in another state, there was the problem of the countries in which there were, yes, many analysts, but all concentrated in a few urban centres within vast territories.

For example, in Argentina, where most analysts reside and work in four cities, Buenos Aires, Córdoba, Mendoza, and Rosario, there are therapists in training who have to travel as much as 400, 500, 600 kilometres to do analysis; nominally they live in a nation where there are many analysts, but in fact they live very far away from them.

The IPA has repeatedly been quite flexible about these alternate analytic settings. Nowadays it would not be so flexible towards (and consequently neither would the SPI even today, for consistency's sake) towards an analysand who living in Mestre could reach the analyst 150 kilometres away: and rightly so, since I could. Certainly, it would have been more difficult for someone from, for example, Bolzano (where there are no analysts in the Society) or other cities and provinces very far from the training centres.

Entire regions of Italy have had to wait a long time to have the first analysts in-house: I am thinking of Puglia, for example. For some years now there have been some in Abruzzo, but the extension outside the large centres has necessarily been gradual and is still limited, given the difficulty of accessing high-frequency training analysis.

Moreover, even in nations with a great psychoanalytic tradition, first and foremost in Great Britain, the problem of the distribution of analysts over the territory is very much felt, with the result that the concentration of colleagues near the training institutes is highest. It is no accident that almost all of them live in London.

I do not want to dwell on this further; I just wanted to evidence that this issue has always been very much alive in the international community.

The SPI, from this point of view, has experienced a fairly extensive and balanced development. There are fourteen Psychoanalytic Centres with about a thousand analysts, in the various regions, and four Training Institutes of the Society.

This kind of articulated societal structure is also present in Germany, whereas this was not the case, for a long time, in France, where most analysts gathered around Paris and Lyon; only then came Toulouse, Bordeaux, and Nice, but the distribution over the territory still remains less than here, although it is gradually changing, as in Spain for that matter.

LN: Your answer makes it clear how even dreams, even when set out by institutions, must be transformed into political projects long term, made up of goals, resources, compromises, partial results.

And then come the unexpected events, such as the pandemic, with its load of heavy restrictions, which disrupted everything.

All analysts have wondered, perforce, about the sudden shift to networking, a mode that has affected so many other professionals as well, I think of teachers and distance education in schools … How has your experience been with this sudden change?

SB: I would say the most appropriate adjective is "traumatic". Just as the outbreak of the pandemic was traumatic, so was the technical revolution that was imposed on us, as soon as we absolutely understood that this was certainly not going to be over in two weeks. At that point, in an earthquake-like, almost war-like climate, a small fraction of analysts in Italy, and I think the same in other countries, continued to see patients in person. Most colleagues, on the other hand, frightened and ultimately also empowered by the situation, decided to work remotely. Ninety-five per cent of them (I don't think I am far wrong in the numbers) had never done it, and had no real experience with it.

I myself had never practised online analysis or psychotherapy before, so I was coming in completely unaware. The only thing I had experienced, but well before the pandemic, had been a series of supervised foreign analysts (North American, Turkish, and Iranian), but they were exceptional situations, and in any case they were not analysis.

Almost all of us, in this circumstance, discovered ourselves to be amateurs at the drop of a hat, operating as we could, at first with a sense of emergency. Having realised after a short time that things were going to go on for a long time, we set ourselves the goal of not abandoning patients and also trying to ensure that in the months ahead we would have sufficient continuity to survive professionally.

LN: And how did you equip yourself to see or hear patients at a distance?

SB: I tried to maintain setting conditions as similar as possible to those to which the patients and I were accustomed, having in mind the principle of "unity of time and place": all my psychotherapy patients that I met face-to-face I saw them on video, taking care to keep the same framing, replaying what they used to see when they sat in front of me, with the bookcase behind the desk standing between us. This was as much as could be done for the "frontiersmen", as I called them.

In contrast, as for the patients who were only lying on the couch, we decided to maintain a lying position mostly on the couch at home, with some adaptive effort and with the almost constant extraordinary partici-pation of dogs and cats, which were soon accepted into sessions as they insisted on being in front of the camera; and I have to say that, to my surprise, the cats turned out to be much more intrusive and intolerant than the dogs, placing themselves often and willingly in front of the camera.

LN: As the restrictions were loosened and the pandemic gradually abated, it was possible to resume the work in presence, each in its own time and manner, and begin to reflect on the experience. More than a year later, what can you say you have learned?

SB: I think I have learned a lot about the dynamics of interpsychic syntonisation, and I have witnessed absolutely significant analytical developments even in remote situations. This was not the case in the very early days, when it was required acclimatisation to learn how to work together in such a novel situation.

In retrospect, I do not take responsibility for determining how far in-presence or remote analysis can be equivalent, nor do I feel I can say that they are the same thing; but I do feel I can testify that even remotely, profound processes happen, effective exchanges take place, and interpretations hit the mark, in a mutual work of contact and mutual comprehension that has impressed me quite a bit.

There has been so much talk over the past two years about direct sensorial aspects, and usually the talk fell on olfactory ones, which are the most blatantly absent remotely. To tell the truth, on certain occasions I even had the impression that colleagues who were so insistent on this lack were exaggerating a bit; I perhaps gave even more importance to voice and words, to the atmospheres that were created from afar.

Of course, there was a lack of the kind of closeness that there is in person, but I think a reflection by Paolo Fonda, who has a great deal of experience in distance analysis and supervision, since he has worked for thirty years with colleagues in some Eastern countries, comes back well. He wondered, with a cautious suspension of judgement, how we can exclude the possibility that certain senses (in this case sight, but also hearing) do not specialise a little at a time and are not accentuated in such a setting, in a compensatory process resulting from the change of conditions.

LN: I feel in full agreement with Fonda's words. Every technical and technological change is accompanied, understandably, by ambivalent reactions, especially on the part of those who have grown up and become familiar and competent with traditional instruments.

As one gets used to the new tools, one can grasp their innovative aspects, which challenge preceding ideas. The senses, precisely, we do not stop using them, but we adopt them differently. The same goes for the body, which is not there, but is there.

For this very reason, I wonder if we should not implement our training with the deeper study of online communication.

SB: I would see well an integration of training with specific courses on this topic, because there are specialised aspects in the clinical use of new technologies.

Methodology, technique, criteria for adjustment with respect to in-person treatment should be taught. I also believe that, from the clinical point of view, there are interesting problems that have not been given much thought to so far.

During a supervision I happened to do at a conference in the United States, I was presented with a clinical situation that in the future might become quite typical: it involved a patient who lived some thirty kilometres (thus a distance that was far from abysmal) from the analyst's office, and who at some point began to ask to be allowed to have online sessions without any particular motive or impediment, but rather "on inspiration", so to speak.

As my colleague began to explain this situation, I was reminded of a patient who years ago had asked to be able to do an analysis with one session per week in person and two remotely; this patient lived and worked in Pieve di Cadore, suffered from a rather serious neurosis, and his request might have made sense. In fact, I sent him to a more accessible colleague from Veneto, and then I heard nothing more about it.

As I listened to the American colleague's account, I gradually realised that the comparison between the two situations did not hold up at all: no, this patient of his would get up in the morning and, at his leisure, inform the analyst that he was going to make the connection instead of coming in. The clinical material showed that there were obvious resistance aspects to his internal and external disposition. The online sessions had little to do with a methodological agreement established as a setting by that analytic couple from the beginning, or from a certain point onward, in a fairly agreed upon way and stable: the patient dodged the session in person for motives that emerged in the material with disarming clarity. What struck me was not that the patient, like everyone else—including us when we were patients—was studying them all, unconsciously, to resist and to defer analytic steps. Instead, it struck me that the analyst did not realise this; that did surprise me, because it would have been part of the job to observe that on that certain day, not scheduled as a remote session, the patient would deflect from the in-person presence and keep away from the analyst, in a situation that was not so arranged.

This is one of many possible examples of how much there is still to define, as well as to study, about these new modes of setting, examining different situations case by case, without accepting or dismissing them out of hand.

LN: One cannot put the toothpaste back into the tube. By now, the dimension of online encounters, whether organisational, educational, or, as in our case, clinical, is part of people's everyday lives, and there is no doubt that this is how it will remain even at the end of the pandemic. One wonders how far analysts, as a community rather than taken individually, will welcome these new modes of encounter without rejecting them outright as transient emergent states.

SB: I respond to you with an association about another patient who lived far away, in an area without analysts.

Early in my career, about forty years ago, I was living and working in the Veneto region, when a fellow came to me for a time from Tarvisi. I don't know if you have any idea where that is.

LN: Google Maps tells me it's 215 kilometres from Mestre, that's almost two and a half hours drive, if we leave now.

SB: Here, this gentleman would take his car and come twice a week to Mestre where I was staying, which was the closest analyst. Otherwise, there was Trieste, but he, for some reason, would come more willingly to me.

Looking back on it today, maybe there had been a chance to work online with the poor guy, who needed it and even had some benefit from the treatment, but who spent two and a half years of hell and risk on the road. In situations like that, why not offer that possibility?

Of course, if, on the other hand, there is someone who lives on the other side of my town and raises his eyebrows at the idea of taking a thirty-minute walk to come here, then the meaning of his reluctance is entirely different …

I think that in the future we will certainly broaden our view of things in this area. One point is that of the sustainability of the analysis project, a topic that I have always been very careful about during the initial proposal and contract phases of a treatment.

When I was operating in my IPA role, in all the nations I visited I would ask how much the sessions cost on average and what the average travel times were for local distances; and I quickly got the idea that there were huge differences, both economically and in the travel required.

These elements are certainly not the only ones that are important or true, but there are also these, and if we think that people can avail themselves of analysis or analytical psychotherapy because they need it, we also need to think realistically about what they can afford, what adaptations or labours or expenses they will be able to undergo; an old Emilian proverb admonishes, "When the road is long, even the straw is heavy …"

I believe that, from the point of view of professional practice, there will be great developments and transformations, due as much to changes in living conditions and mentality as to new technologies, which will surprise us. I cannot say how, when and how profoundly, but I see it as a natural progress, no doubt about it.

LN: Speaking of future developments, do you have a suggestion for those who are starting our profession?

SB: My suggestion is only one, and that is that this profession cannot be done in half, with one foot in one boat and the other in another. I am not saying that one cannot work in public service as well; that is another matter.

I am talking about internal, deep identity: if one is an analyst, one should become an analyst, and one should be an analyst.

This means so many things: to have care and awareness of the relationship with oneself, of the relationship with the other, of the now far more than secular culture that founds our professional history, that is part of us.

In short, let him or her not delude himself or herself into thinking that he or she can do "also" or "a little", the analyst, or that he or she can also do so many other things that have nothing to do with analysis or that conflict with it. The analyst has to really do it, otherwise it's better that he or she doesn't do it.

LN: I have one last question about training. Analytic training is based on three training pillars: the experiential pillar of personal analysis, the didactic pillar of seminars and clinical courses, and the pillar of supervision of one's own analytic work, which you also told us about.

This is a very thorough, often decennial training, centred on the individual analyst and his or her deep relationship with the patient. In recent decades, however, there has been a lack in group and institutional work, to the point that a very evocative term has been coined, which you are familiar with: the "Fourth Pillar". A term much used in assembl'es and conferences, but I'm afraid still unused elsewhere. What is it about?

SB: I am familiar with that term because I created it. It is the flour of my own sack.

We analysts are part of a professional and scientific community, and above all, beyond the external structural aspects, we experience within ourselves a world of presences and interlocutors. They are, first of all, our analytic family, of which we have already spoken, then they are the various colleagues in a more extended sense: they are the course mates we bring in from our training, and they are the colleagues of the Centre or Institute to which we adhere for the rest of our lives.

All of them we "carry" in various ways: in a persecutory way when we fear our own inadequacies or the criticism of others; in a deeply interesting way when we can imagine and really dialogue with them even within ourselves (what would he say and what would she say in a certain work situation, in front of a certain problem?).

These internal interlocutors are part of us. They also structure us, organise us. In the really good cases of our developmental experience, they become creative interlocutors: when our training has reached a level of sufficient maturity we consult them, but then we decide.

How do we consult them? Through a fairly free-flowing preconscious frequentation, we let them come to mind; it is the internal coexistence with these familiar objects that enrich our professional lives.

It is always said that an analyst to be such must have at least one patient and at least one colleague: I think this is very true.

The Fourth Pillar, as I have understood it (other colleagues have developed it in another sense), is the progressive acquisition of the ability, and also the pleasure, of working together with others, of exchanging with others.

This ability could be elicited and coached as early as during training, within preorganised moments in which clinical material is handled among colleagues of equal experience, all of whom are learners, without a supervisor present.

Of course, supervisors are needed, and there are the classic institutional situations in which trainees work with them, individually and also in groups; but there would also need to be occasions in which candidates can discuss the material with each other.

This is already happening, appropriately but unfortunately in a limited way, in IPSO (the International Organisation of Analysts in Training), whereas for me those experiences should be a structural part of the training: they train in the pleasure of working together with colleagues throughout one's professional life, without having to depend always and only on parental or parental figures.

We could compare this experiential phase to the enjoyment of playing in the backyard with friends.

The danger to be avoided is the subsequent isolation of the professional once the training is over, and the best antidote towards that danger is to have accustomed the professional, from a young age, to finding stimulation and satisfaction in clinical dialogue with his colleagues.

This is the philosophy of the Fourth Pillar of training.

CHAPTER 10

Rough questions

LN: Among the notes I had prepared for our meeting, a few specific questions remained at the back that I would call "rough" in some cases.

The first concerns the different forms of sexuality that are emerging with fewer inhibitions and less shame than in the past. At the same time, however, in a world where pornography is rampant and sex seems to have been cleared through customs in all its forms, we are faced with taboos, obstacles, and even violent rejections of forms of sexuality that disturb the "quiet life". On television, on billboards, not to mention sex videos, women are deprived of all modesty, yet breastfeeding in public still causes scandal. Gay couples, who have struggled out of a state of almost associated clandestinity, are "erased" from the regulations of many states and suffer the punches of the gangs of kids who attack them every day.

I wonder if this apparent tangle of contradictions also has to do with the rejection of otherness: sex, yes, but only as I say.

SB: I believe that even in the vast area of sexuality and related collective phantasmatic* experience there are complex realities in motion and transformation, but I also believe that things proceed less linearly than one imagines and would like.

As is the case with all major evolutions, the recognition and acceptance of different, relationally good, but new forms of sexuality take time.

For example, the fact that a homosexual couple can be respected and recognised in its valid relational ways—what would be the natural outcome of today's consciousness-raising—may, however, encounter two obstacles. On the one hand, it may clash against the inevitable resistance of the common mentality to accept that there are sexual orientations other than the traditional and conventional ones; on the other hand, it may stimulate, vice versa, a façade conformism in exhibiting ideological acceptance, regardless, of sexual orientations and forms of relationship, the real quality of which is unknown.

In fact, there are sadomasochistic and more or less openly destructive relationships as much among heterosexuals as among homosexuals, and the criterion of whether or not to value couples on the basis of orientation *per se* alone should not be absolute and generalised.

I believe that psychoanalysis plays a valuable role in this, because it can help to recognise the intrinsic and substantive quality of human relationships: creative, respectful, appreciative, and affective relationships can arise in any form of sexual orientation, whilst other relationships can be deeply destructive, sadomasochistic, or hyper-dependent, regardless of the identities and orientations involved. The most mature analytic attitude would be not to idealise or stigmatise anything *a priori*, and instead to explore—quietly and without prejudice—the substantive quality of relationships.

LN: Given your answer, I feel like touching, in this conversation of ours, on a very painful but little-known aspect that closely concerns the SPI, to which we both belong. In Italy, the first openly homosexual candidates have only been accepted into training since the 2000s. Before that, they were discarded *a priori*. This is just one example of how psychoanalysis, through its institutions, has neglected the affective quality of relationships, which we have just talked about.

From a certain point of view, the theories of fixations to the pregenital stages, needless to mention the anal stage, represented a very severe form of judgement, or prejudice. I thought that leaving a written record of this silent discrimination might be helpful in raising awareness of this issue.

You, who have had your eye on the SPI and IPA in recent decades, can you tell us something about the topic?

SB: I became a training analyst in 1998, and later also a selector. Shortly after 2000, in one of the first selections I attended as an examiner, I met a would-be candidate who explicitly stated his orientation.

I explored with interest and care his relational world, which developed further through analysis. I then discovered that the other two selectors were of the same conviction as I was, that is, they shared the view that the aspirant had a very, very good quality of relating to others; therefore, I had no hesitation in formulating a positive opinion: he was a person who, by accessing the training, would do good not only to himself, but also to the patients with whom he would work, and to the colleagues with whom he would interact and collaborate.

I was glad of this conviction later, because it was confirmed to me, as far as what little I knew about this colleague's professional development. A similar thing happened shortly thereafter with another aspirant.

Of course, I would not have expressed the same opinion, neither regarding a homosexual person, nor regarding a heterosexual person, if I had found, in the quality of their object relations, serious disturbances, serious distortions, malfunctions such as to prevent them from interacting in an adequate manner with a patient.

I am convinced that there is a non-dissociated and indeed very substantial continuity between personal object relations and professional object relations, there is a continuum. If a person seems—or poses to seem—very harmonious in the professional field and is not so on a personal or vice versa level, in my opinion there is something to be reviewed analytically, in depth.

The big news in the 2000s was the acceptance that the quality of internal and external object relations was considered the essential discriminating factor in the selection of potential analysts.

LN: And in the IPA, what was it able to ascertain?

SB: What happened in the IPA is that the Committee on Gender Diversities, which was created during my presidency, has seen very good growth. It has organised a great number of scientific events, but above all it has opened up the community mindset by developing an attitude of research, investigation, and exploration on various sexualities, therefore also on heterosexualities (plural), that was not there before.

For the IPA, I just participated in a selection of papers on the topic of Gender Diversities and I found studies of an extraordinary quality, both on homosexuality, transsexuality, and all the developments, processes, evolutions that human sexuality in a general sense can know. The concept of perversion is not lost, but it should be individuated and limited to a set of characteristics and links in which the quality of object relations is unhealthy.

Conversely, the profound naturalness of certain developments can be recognised precisely by the good quality of the object relationship. From this point of view there has been an evolution, first of all scientific, of enormous importance, broadening of horizons and also of different institutional organisations. However, this does not mean accepting everything as valid and sound, because we have become much more competent in recognising and evaluating, precisely, relational quality.

LN: The idea of not dedicating this book only to analysts, but to broaden the audience to curious people, is part of my way of looking at our subject. I love the idea of "bringing the plague", as Freud said when he was about to land in the United States for a series of lectures. Yet, it always seems that analysts do not dialogue enough with society and institutions. In what way, do you think, should we position ourselves, so as not to appear as all-rounders dissertating everything from their comfortable armchair? In short, to be credible.

SB: I suspect that quite a few clichés thrive on this issue.

Every now and then there is a campaign from some analysts along the lines of, "It is good for analysts to come out of their ivory tower". I have to laugh because this sounds like a decision that is up to analysts, when it is not.

First, analysts have a way of conducting themselves, in their speech, that is not very compatible (often not at all compatible) with the speed of contemporary communication. We analysts reflect, think, before responding; we do not like catch-phrases, which risk becoming simplistic; we tend to analyse things in a complex way, in depth. All this is not compatible with the fast pace of media exchange. The way of speaking of an analyst usually arouses a sense of impatience with the hurried television and radiophonic interviewers, who work in spots, in one-liners, who do not tolerate pauses and thoughtfulness.

The analyst, when he or she speaks, brings with him or her a world of thoughts and a wealth of experience from which he or she does not dissociate, and indeed consults at least a little when speaking.

Other professionals, who do not have the same familiarity with this deep internal contact, travel freely and quietly "without carry-on baggage", and thus appear much quicker and more effective in their interventions.

As an example of this, I always cite philosophers: they have a speed of communication commensurate with the fact that they can proceed conceptually, without necessarily having to consult the whole experiential and affective self; as an analyst tends to do.

This is also true for certain psychologists or psychiatrists who go fast and decisive because they are sectional, they have their recurring patterns. Sometimes they are sharper precisely because of this: they "cut" the object faster and more essentially.

And so far, the considerations I am developing would only seem to enhance the merits—though unacknowledged—of the way analysts function.

However, it must also be admitted, unfortunately, that our interventions are usually verbose, are slow, and that our ability not to refer to one's own jargon, theories, or concepts is poor.

In order to communicate with the outside world, we should speak in a common language, following that criterion of our Bolognese colleague Gino Zucchini, who said he preferred Italian to psychoanalytic. We all agree on this, but it is a difficult task for us, who have spent time within a certain theoretical-technical dictionary and it is not easy for us to translate it into the language of the media.

The SPI had an external press office for many years, we also hired a journalist with many contacts and connections at the editorial offices of newspapers and television stations, but the results were modest.

In short, the psychoanalytic discourse has its own complexity, and from there there is no escape.

People often ask, with despairing reductiveness: "Doctor, what does it mean if one does this, or says that?" expecting an equally quick and hasty answer that we cannot give.

There are occasions that lend themselves better to this, such as the public lectures that you often organise and which I too have had the pleasure of attending twice.

Those were a privileged condition for us, because we knew that we would have a couple of hours to calmly dialogue.

Instead, when I was interviewed by journalists in the print media, or on television, or on the radio, the times were syncopated and beating, and so I tried to adjust to the pace set by the presenters; but it certainly was not my pace, and I know it is the same for most of my colleagues.

LN: Now a question about the relationship between the Italian state and the mental health of its citizens.

The pandemic has seen great voluntary participation of the Order of Psychologists, of many scientific societies, including the SPI, for tens of thousands of free telephone consultations. It is certainly a meritorious operation, but what I wonder is, whether volunteering does not testify to the resignation of psychologists to the fact that institutions, administrations, and politics do not intend to take on the costs of mental health for citizens.

In addition, fellow analysts working in the national healthcare system, both psychologists and psychiatrists, complain about the scarcity of resources that has all but wiped out the supply of psychotherapy. The intake of patients is mandatory, so each of them is responsible for 200, 300, 400 patients. It is inevitable that for many of them, the work can only be limited to psychodiagnostic consultations, possible pharmacological support, especially for severe cases of personality disorders and psychosis, or short psychoeducational courses. The relationship with private professionals, at least in our region (Emilia), is slim to none. Comparing myself with colleagues, there seems to be almost a split between private and public service, poor communication. I have witnessed at least three or four cases in which psychiatrists have considered the discontinuation of psychotherapeutic pathways that were working, because in their opinion they were upsetting the patients, or not serving them. Admissions decided without consulting the therapists who had been treating people for years.

Does everyone think for themselves and save themselves?

SB: That's how it is, there's no point in denying it. The economic aspect has something to do with it, but it is also a consequence of a careless mentality that is not very helpful towards the real therapists of mental disorders.

The solutions that have been adopted have been (a) to contract out to families the management of the costs of most mental disorders, and (b) to nominally set up—just to save officialdom and face—services in which an unsustainable and unrealistic demand is poured on psychiatrists and psychologists to deal with.

In the official statements of administrators, who depend on politicians, they describe a wondrous abundance of facilities, services, and care that is not possible, because every health worker can only do so much.

Staffing levels throughout public health have been reduced for budgetary reasons, but what is certain is that, compared to other items of expenditure in the sector, mental health is absolutely undersized.

It is an unrealistic saving as this ultimately leads to other issues, because patients who are not sufficiently treated and cared for then cost in so many other respects; they do harm to themselves and others, create very heavy situations of hospitalisation and social care that generate enormous supplementary costs.

There is still a lot of work to be done in this area: the application of pharmacological psychiatry, which has been useful, indeed very useful in some cases, is being unduly extended to a much wider range of conditions that could be treated in other ways.

Psychiatry services and general practitioners prescribe many antidepressants, sometimes even in bereavement situations, where, instead, the accompaniment should be of a different nature, without exciting and turning up the engine speed with Prozac and drugs like that. So, it ends up that physiological bereavements are treated as if they were a pathology.

And I could go on with glaring and tragic examples, such as those of children who are given diagnoses of arousal-hyperactivity syndromes that are too superficial and not very clinically thorough; or many other situations involving minors that are so sad because the possibility of treating them better technically is instead hastily resolved with crude and simplistic protocols.

LN: I pick up on your answer because I would like to emphasise what you are saying: various pathologies or other difficult situations potentially could be addressed with good psychotherapy, instead they are treated with drugs or other solutions.

There are countless situations in which psychotherapy is not prescribed, is not indicated, is not even mentioned. Years ago, I took a very suffering and inhibited young lady in for analysis, who later turned out to be full of resources. In the previous ten years she had had three major depressive crises, for which she had taken several drugs, and never had anyone told her that there was such a thing as psychotherapy.

SB: A temporary solution is too often put in place, which packages the patient and disposes of him or her with a very quick "revolving door" diagnostic-therapeutic dispositive, then sends him or her home compensated pharmacologically. I insist: drugs are useful and sometimes indispensable for certain conditions. Instead, they are used hand over fist, "*a becchime*", in so many cases in which instead they are not at all the elective solution.

LN: People are beginning to talk, at least as a mirage, about the figure of public care psychologist. Or maybe it is only our Order that is talking about it, I don't know. Certainly, it is a fact that primary care physicians are faced with at least 30 per cent of patients who would need a different kind of listening, for which they are not trained.

SB: I am convinced of that; I am certain of that. The idea of a public care psychologist does not seem to me to be bad, if it were developed in a certain way: a kind of counter to which some people, from a certain area or a certain neighbourhood, can turn to begin to make contact with their emotional issues and talk to someone, in a protected way, with a listening free of prejudice. Open listening.

LN: Speaking of prejudice, listening, and dialogue, I have several colleagues from different theoretical orientations, some of whom passionately and profitably practice cognitive-behavioural therapies. There are those who teach mindfulness courses, EMDR is emerging very strongly as a therapy for trauma. These are therapies that thus, at first glance, appear more contemporary.

In the hallways of various scientific conferences, in front of coffee machines, caricatured depictions are wasted on us, the bow-tied wizards, and them treating people like computers to be reprogrammed. Speaking of religious wars ...

You are a great integrator of psychoanalys s. What is your view on the coexistence between psychoanalysis and these other disciplines? Do we continue to coexist and each do their own thing? Maybe some patients are better suited to some therapies, others to others?

SB: I think they are essentially different practices; I'm not going to go out on a limb and say whether they are good or not because I don't know them enough.

Speaking very broadly, I get the idea that there are myriad solutions for different kinds of needs and at different levels of depth: also religious restraint and assistance, militancy in political parties, the practice of meditative disciplines, organised sports cheering, etc. have a useful function for the psychic balance of many pecple. Similar to the formula in vogue today of the "diffuse hotel" in old town centres, we can recognise that there are an infinite number of "diffuse mental health agencies", which are useful but not recognised as such: bars, community centres, voluntary associations, parishes, gyms, and schools of oriental disciplines. And there are endless therapeutic options, quite different from psychoanalysis and its more pertinent derivatives.

Even in psychotherapy, one can seek momentary support, perhaps of a targeted or consultative kind, or treatment of a major and lasting level.

During a trip, some people stop at the service station, without leaving the highway to look for a restaurant; and if one at that moment needs to feel a little better by quickly calming the hunger pangs, the service station is just fine. The service is quick, inexpensive, and one can feed well there as well. On the other hand, if one wishes to have a different gastronomic experience, one will go elsewhere.

Prescribing in-depth analytical treatment to persons who, on balance, have no real need for it is not a good choice, as we said earlier. Similarly, suggesting surface treatments to people who with such limited experience do not have the changes necessary for a good quality of life is not a good practice.

There may be a need for an anaesthetist, there may be a need for a surgeon, there may be a need for an orthopaedist—the levels of intervention vary according to need. We don't send everyone to the surgeon, however, we don't advise someone who has a serious internal affection to go to the beautician.

LN: Recently I have often had to take quick lunches, and there is no more unbearable thing than going to a restaurant in such cases. The waiters are so obsequious, thoughtful, and reflective, and one ends up paying a high bill.

SB: Not only that, in fact, I will confess one thing to you: some of the dishes you find at truck stops I like very much. The fact is that there are different situations, different times, different perspectives. And it is important to distinguish each person's needs.

LN: And we come towards the end. I have kept two issues that are very complex and I hope I am quite clear in expounding them.

We take it for granted that analysis leads to greater freedom to take care of oneself, with fewer pressing constraints dictated by the superego and the Ego Ideal. I was curious to know, in your experience, how analysts work in countries where not only is individual freedom by no means a given, but sometimes being free and independent is not even a value.

I'm thinking of colleagues who live in places like China, and Iran, but also closer to home in Hungary, where the government is putting a lot of constraints on civil liberties. I wanted to understand whether their theoretical approach contradicts the governmental and cultural dictates of those countries, or whether it harmonises with the dominant culture. How is analytic identity configured in such contexts?

I understand that I am making very large generalisations, but I think some food for thought can give us that.

SB: Yes, I really have to say that in this field, more than the risk, there is the certainty of generalisation! However, having known quite from the inside some of these realities (both having talked to colleagues and having been to these places, and having examined in supervision the clinical material produced locally), I have noticed important differences between countries that share authoritarian regimes and sociopolitical atmospheres, but that are characterised by very different underlying cultures.

For example, Iran, where officially there is a ubiquitous and monolithic religious presence, from a perspective of psychoanalytic survey offers a striking picture of a rather split reality: the patients of Iranian analysts are often people belonging to the upper-middle class both culturally and socially, yes, they live in a public regime atmosphere, but they indulge in a much freer private lifestyle than we imagine. There is a surprising open-mindedness in analysts and patients than we would imagine on the basis of our Western clichés. On the basis of the analysis of their clinical material, however, it seemed to me to detect a certain inner dysmetria—I would really call it that—in the current lifestyle of many patients who seem to be in search of a somewhat lost balance; to the point that, at times, one even gets the impression that they suffer from insufficient overall contentment, that they do not show the internalised sense of limitation that there is in other nations, and that they manifest a kind of diffuse imbalance. It's a strange psychosocial phenomenon: the private is ultra-liberated, the public is ultra-limited, and the work of integrating these two so-called realities still appears largely in progress.

On the other hand, I found consequences—which endure to this day—of great inhibitory limitation and conditioning in contact with deep emotional life in some clinical material presented by colleagues from Poland: in certain cases, one can perceive—in a watermark, rather than in a manifest way—the transgenerational presence of many internal occlusions originating from the previous ways of life under the communist regime, which still persist today in an internalised and unconscious way. I have been able to see that the work of Polish colleagues is consequently very much oriented towards the recovery of greater psychic freedom and towards the reappropriation of a sense of subjectivity and individuality in many of their patients.

The sense of subjectivity is the new frontier that Chinese colleagues also seem to be working with today. The government, in the face of still very authoritarian and very closed aspects, seems to have rediscovered its value, in conjunction with an interesting change in the sociocultural atmosphere (among other things, they recently lifted the ban on having a third child).

The Chinese government is allowing the spread of psychoanalysis, albeit with some caution. It keeps it partially in check by encouraging its development, especially in academia: many of China's new analysts are also university professors. Nevertheless, the recuperation of subjectivity is really a work in progress. After generations in which the subject was hardly supposed to exist, in favour mainly or exclusively of the community, the individual is making a comeback in the Chinese mindset.

In the more advanced countries of Eastern Europe today, such as those of the former Yugoslavia, analysts are living quite well operationally and functionally, because a discrete, undercurrent process of progressive cultural openness is unfolding in Slovenia, Bosnia, and Serbia.

You mentioned Hungary, where a hyper-traditionalist and rather restrictive political regime is in place, but which is also endowed with a very strong and rich psychoanalytic tradition: the Hungarian Psychoanalytic Society has existed since the time of Ferenczi—that is, since the beginning of the twentieth century—and has a great heritage of analytic history and culture, and seems to have a theoretical and operational base that is little affected by the political-cultural trend of the moment. We can be quite comfortable, so to speak, because Hungarian analysts enjoy solid multigenerational roots and have strong identity originality.

Another interesting change, which I would like to point out, is the fact that analysts of colour are increasing, whether in the United States, Brazil, or South Africa, with original contributions of great quality.

Still regarding the originality of what is being produced in our scientific field, I have found the contributions of Japanese colleagues extremely interesting. Japan hosts one of the oldest psychoanalytic societies in the IPA, but it has a limited number of analysts because Japanese society is extremely selective. They produce papers of enormous interest: I was able to listen to three or four of them live and they seemed special, of impressive depth, in harmony with their centuries-old philosophic and aesthetic tradition. It is a world for us to discover.

CHAPTER 11

The end of the world

LN: I conclude our conversation with a series of reflections on today's world, or rather, on what seems to be the end of the world, if you will allow me the expression.

For some time now I have been experiencing feelings of unease, of restlessness, of fear for the future, which I struggle to communicate. I find myself wondering whether my daughter will live in a poorer country, whether she will have to emigrate abroad, whether the house I am buying today with my sacrifices will be worth anything. Will the polar bears I see in documentaries still exist?

I know I have a depressive undercurrent that I have been carrying around for a lifetime, but last night something happened that stayed with me. I was preparing with my colleague and friend, Anna Cordioli, for this conversation of ours, when point-blank she said to me, "We analysts need to start talking about the end of the world … It's like I feel like I'm on top of a big pimple about to burst. This is Western civilisation".

I thought about that. International politics no longer provides such stability. For some months now, the clock of history has seemed to turn back: the Cold War, tanks in Europe, the Taliban takeover in Afghanistan, and before that the Islamic State in Syria. The semblance of order of the past decades is crumbling.

For the past couple of years, unless one lives in a refrigerator, no one can deny that the planet is burning. The summer just past was among the hottest ever, and some murmur that it is among the coolest compared to those to come. In 2000, we were 6 billion people; twenty years on, we are 8 billion. And let's not talk about the pandemic: in a few short years, it caused a kind of global revolution. We are still unsure whether we will return to normal or if now live in a new normal.

Now I ask you, somewhat provocatively, whether psychoanalysts are not on average too old to fully experience the restlessness of the world over the next thirty years, or whether, like all other people, they realise the danger only when they are very close to it and therefore have a hard time seeing that Western society as we know it, and the world more generally, is facing terrifying changes.

SB: I share that view to a certain extent, and I tell you among other things that the denial capacity of analysts is sometimes impressive.

We have a glaring historical example of this: Freud was almost forced to leave Vienna by the insistence of a good part of his colleagues from other nations, because all in all he did not recognise the magnitude, the magnitude of what was not only about to be unleashed, but was already visibly underway. Caught up in his routine, his affections, his quiet bourgeois habits in Berggasse, he struggled to fully accept the idea that a mass extermination was underway that was destined in a very short time to endanger him and his loved ones. They had to push him away.

This is an interesting example of what can prevent analysts, even the most forewarned or disenchanted, from recognising major epochal changes. Climate change today is recognised by all analysts, unanimously agreeing that it is a major collective problem, dramatic in its own right, but with psychological side effects as well: denial and denial, as the case may be. As recently as ten years ago, Sally Weintrobe (2013), a British colleague, wrote, along with other British society analysts, a seminal book on the reasons for collective resistance to acknowledging dramatic climate change.

Regarding the problem of overpopulation, on the other hand, there has been a censorship, a blindness, a scotoma[6] particularly in our field as well: to think that there are too many of us—the old Malthusian hypothesis that many thinkers are, by the way, re-evaluating

---

[6] Defect in the visual field relating to a more or less extensive area where black or coloured, sometimes glittering, spots appear, due to lesion of the optic pathways.

as realistic—would undermine an ideal image of analysts as "good" thinkers. Perhaps it sounds like an overly bold recognition, bordering on impiety, effusive towards not only current morality, but even the general feeling of inter-human solidarity: which is true, because it is certainly not good-brotherly thinking to think that there are too many children.

It is equally true, however, that this thought is emerging, albeit amidst a thousand conflicts; and if democracy and the equidistributive mentality, in spite of everything, continue to advance in the world, this will mean that all these "too many" will rightly have to have the same consumer's rights: and thus will in turn produce carbon dioxide, waste, cementing, and further needs to be met. After all, who could deny that it is ethically and politically right that everyone, to the extent possible, can equally have it all, do it all, and go everywhere, as hitherto granted only to a privileged section of the population? And is it equally "right" (again in terms of collective ethical sentiment) that the procreative capacity of human beings is not be restricted: who would dare say anything against it?

This, however, may prospect an overburdened world in short order, in spite of the philosophical and political correctness of the principles of social equity, and the denial of this complex and painful reality could in turn lead to future scenarios of an unbelievably tragic nature.

We might ask then: if psychoanalysts, albeit somewhat belatedly, have finally produced important observations on the issue of pathologic psychic defences induced by the climate problem, and conversely almost nothing with respect to the demographic issue, is it not precisely because they fear that a reflection on the latter would prove even more dangerous and offensive to the depurated and uplifting image we have of ourselves, and because it would bring into play painful and psychologically undefendable anti-ethical and anti-social phantasms?

In the face of this complexity, one realises that the risk of moving towards a less liveable world is there. New generations realise this more, those who have children think about it.

LN: Do you remember the song "The Old Man and the Child" (*Il vecchio e il bambino*)? Francesco Guccini, 30 years old, gave a glimpse of a world that is too much approaching.

Associations?

SB: My first association is to the flight from Kabul in the imminence of the arrival of the Taliban, to the dramatic television images of the thousands of people who would have wanted to leave, but there were only a certain number of planes, so capacity was limited, no matter how admirable the forces put in place.

This scene condensed into an image of what we then saw happening again in Ukraine, with images of fleeing people crowding onto the few available trains: it could be the drama of the future and it is already the drama of the present.

There are many of us, too many of us; the anthropisation of the planet is extensive, the cementing of green areas is rife. Emissions serve to enable a fairly egalitarian standard of living for the great masses—who could say that's not fair? However, it is increasingly difficult to give everyone and allow everyone to enjoy the same goods, services, and opportunities if the population grows at the current rate.

There were 50.2 million Italians in 1960; they became 59.5 million in 2020. Thus, the population has grown, but not so much, proportionally, as to justify the level of pollution solely on the basis of the number of citizens: rather, the problem is the change in living habits.

Until the late 1950s, before the real economic boom, 70 per cent of Italians, roughly, lived in the countryside and had a high level of residency and settledness, as well as a very low level of consumption. People stayed more or less on the farm where they worked and once a week went to the neighbouring village where there was a market. Since then, people's movement and consumption has increased much more; the latest generation do many more things and go to many more places than they used to. This figure gives an idea of the complexity of the problem and future prospects.

LN: With these sour notes …

SB: Yes, sour ones …

LN: … we have reached the end of our journey. In thanking you for your generosity in indulging my curiosity, I ask how you want to end this conversation of ours. I leave you the last word.

SB: The last word is "sustainable". It is a word that I would apply not only to ecology, economics, politics, and sociality in general, but also to psychoanalysis.

Sustainability, that is, a realistic recognition of what people can really ask of psychoanalysis and what we psychoanalysts can actually offer, do, support, ask for, will be a crucial issue for our work in the future.

Psychoanalysis will evolve by seeking a sustainability of its actual practice and what can be done, on a basis that will have to hold together—we don't know what we wish to do, what we should do, and what we can do.

This is the old schema that Dr Molinari taught me, which was very simple and said that the Central Ego can ask itself: what do I wish to do? What can I do? What do I need to do? Combined, these three questions can lead to the What do I want to do?: which is not the simple desire, but what I consciously and responsibly decide after exploring and weighing the dimensions of the ideal, the ought, and the possible.

It is a grid that remains most interesting because it brings together the different sides of psychopathology: the problem of neurosis in those who do not know what they want; the aspects of psychosis in those who do not know what they can realistically do, because they cultivate omnipotence; and the potential aspects of perversion in those who do not respect what they have to do.

The person sufficiently capable of thinking, eventually decides, based on these three parameters, what his will and—hopefully—the course of his actions will be.

I believe that psychoanalysis in the future will come to terms with what it wants, what it can and what it must do. So, it will have to balance the ideal with the mandate of duty and the recognition of limits and possibilities.

A blow to our residual, unconfessed, omnipotent ambitions.

A bitter pill to swallow, but also a decidedly healthy dietary measure.

Glossary

Abstinence
The regimen in which psychoanalysis takes place, which involves abstaining as much as possible from the satisfaction of desires through actions or behaviour. This encourages the expression of these through speech and free associations.

Acting out
The action that replaces thought which constitutes an impulsive discharge of emotional tension.

Container (psychic)
The mental structure is capable of receiving, housing, developing, and transforming psychic contents, i.e. affects and thoughts. The proper functioning of the container is a requirement for mental health; its malfunctions and/or ruptures lead to the most serious mental pathologies, personality disorders, and psychosis, respectively.

Countertransference

This is the psychological reaction of the analyst (or other people) to the transference to which he or she is subjected. Depending on the theoretical models to which the analyst refers, it can be seen as either hindering or helping the therapeutic process.

Defence (mechanisms of)

These are automatic, mostly unconscious processes by which the mind protects itself from anguish. Some examples are removal, regression, projection, and dissociation.

Denial

In denial we think or say that a certain thing is not so, when in fact it is (e.g. I am not old, when in fact I am). In denial, we don't think that a thing is not so, we simply don't think about it at all, and we bypass the problem without consideration.

Dissociation

Defensive mechanism consisting of compartmentalisation of experience. Dissociations can be functional when they facilitate complex mental tasks, whilst they are dysfunctional when they are responsible for dissociative disorders.

Drives

The psychosomatic impulses that cause tension in the organism, which demands satisfaction. The main ones are the sexual and self-preservation drives and the destructive or self-destructive drives.

Ego

One of the three psychic instances according to Freud, along with the id and the superego. It is the structure charged with the integration of needs, desires, moral demands and the limits of external reality. It is responsible for cognitive abilities and psychic defenses.

Egosyntonic

A symptom that is not recognised as such, thus disturbing (i.e. egodystonic), but is considered by the patient to be a functional part of the self. Examples include hallucinations and delusions during psychotic crises.

Empathy
Empathy is generally regarded as one's ability to empathise with other people, to feel or sense their states of mind. Psychoanalytic empathy is a more specific and complex phenomenon concerned with getting in touch with a wider range of the patient's emotions, both those he or she experiences and those that are removed or split off.

Enactment
A clinical concept according to which the analyst and patient act out in external reality a script that they are not yet able to psychically represent and verbally communicate to themselves. The analyst, at a later time, can retrieve the meaning of the acted exchange and share it with the patient.

Fixation
Locking of libido to a certain object of satisfaction, or similar to an organisation related to a certain developmental stage.

Free association
The method of free association, developed by Freud, consists of letting one's thoughts take free course, trying not to judge, censor, or direct them somewhere specific.

Grandiose self
An archaic state of the infantile self that manifests itself in the form of grandiose ambitions and fantasies. The Grandiose Self is an absolute narcissistic dimension in which all attention is focused on the self.

Hallucinate/hallucination
Hallucination is a subjective perception, which does not correspond to stimulation by sense organs (hearing voices or sounds that do not exist, for example). It is physiological in early infantile development, as the birth of thought (breast hallucination when the mother is not present), whilst later it is present in acute and special emotional situations, in psychotic pathologies, or other states of illness or intoxication.

Hypomanic regime
A behavioural style characterised by continuous arousal, aimed at avoiding depressive feelings and thoughts.

Idealisation
A psychic mechanism of bringing the characteristics of an object to perfection. It is a fairly primitive system because it districts the representation of reality.

Impulses
See **Drives**.

Internal world
The set of thoughts and feelings that populate an individual's mind. It is spoken of as opposed to the external world, as objective reality is defined. Clearly, this is a polarity utilised to simplify a much more nuanced continuum.

Interpsychic
The interpsychic is the equivalent of the healthy and necessary fusion conditions and processes that in nature enable vital (nurturing, nurturing, regulatory) exchanges between human beings in the early stages of life and growth (see also pp. 85–86 in Chapter 6). The interpsychic is an occasional and natural mode of co-experience and collaboration connecting two individuals, and not a structural and stable condition. It does not necessarily imply that a person or subject is present. As a prototype of this, when a mother breastfeeds a baby at the beginning there is no overt personal status, but rather there is a natural cooperation between mouth and nipple that allows the mother and baby to "collaborate" in a regime of good fusion cooperation. The two are able to exchange internal content (both physical and emotional) through their specific organs, entering and leaving the internal world (Bolognini, 2008). These bodily relations, initially experienced with a low level of mentalisation but with a high degree of imprinting, will function as subsequent intrapsychic equivalents mainly at a

preconscious level (as occurs e.g. in most cases in creative processes). See also **Transpsychic** or **Intrapsychic**.

Intersubjective and interpersonal

Concepts in some cases, but not always, overlap and are interchangeable with each other and with interpsychic. The difference is based on the fact that a subject is a human being with a sufficiently coherent core of contact with the self, capable of experiencing his or her own emotions with a good sense of self-continuity. There may be a cohesive and sufficiently intense perception of one's self, even if the process of separation is not complete and personal boundaries are still poorly defined (e.g. many artists are strongly subjective despite a low definition—at least partially—of their boundaries as persons). A person, on the other hand, is a human being with a well-defined identity and bodily and psychic boundaries in his or her self-representation, and with a psychic distinction from the other sufficiently clear. A relevant part of his or her well-differentiated mental activity can be developed at a conscious level, obviously with the problems and defences that have been explored by psychoanalysis; nevertheless, a person can be defined as such even if he or she has tenuous contact with his or her own subjectivity, as is described in many pathological cases. Because of this, "being a subject" is not always equivalent to "being a person", and vice versa: one condition does not exclude the other, but neither does it imply it.

Intrapsychic

Related to within the psyche of an individual.

Kleinian school

The psychoanalytic movement inspired by the theories of the prominent British psychoanalyst Melanie Klein, according to which children develop unconscious fantasies early on about their relationship with their mother's body. Some of these fantasies provoke anguish, which can be reduced by interpreting them, thus making the patient aware of them.

Libido

Freud calls libido the psychic, emotional energy that the individual invests in the objects that excite and interest him or her, and withdraws when the investment wanes or is extinguished. But it is also the psychic equivalent of the subsequent intimate interactions that at all stages of life, including adult life, make possible the natural, fluctuating, non-pathological passage of content from someone's interior to someone else's interior: in sexuality, in learning, in the complexities of development.

Masochism

A set of concepts describing the turning of sadism, on a sexual level or more generally on a moral level, against oneself.

Mentalization

Mental imagery activity that allows people's behaviours to be interpreted as the outcome of internal mental states i.e. the result of desires, expectations, needs, thoughts, and feelings. According to Bateman and Fonagy (2016), a mentalization-based therapy aims to help patients understand their own and others' mental functioning, and is particularly indicated for personality disorders.

Metapsychology

The set of theories of the psyche developed by Freud.

Metasetting

The system of rules, norms, and expectations shared by society that co-constitute the implicit framework for living. For example, the analyst has a practice, acts as a professional, and is dressed in a manner appropriate to the local culture.

Narcissism

This is a term that refers to several psychological and psychoanalytical concepts, which make reference to the privileged relationship with oneself over others. A certain amount of narcissism is necessary for the maintenance of self-esteem and a good relationship with oneself, whilst pathological forms lead to rigid, continuous and real feelings, thoughts and behaviours of inferiority or superiority.

Narcissistically mirroring/twin relationship

A relationship in which the object is not fully recognised as such, thus distinct from self, but is experienced as its own alter ego, a figure more like itself than it actually is.

Negation
See **Denial**.

Neurosis

A state of the psyche that is guaranteed to be well contained, which is the seat of conflicts between different needs and desires. These conflicts and the ways of handling them give rise to individual personality or neurotic forms of suffering (obsessions, phobias, etc.). When the container is deficient we speak of psychosis, that is, situations in which external and internal realities can blur together, causing delusions and hallucinations. In the middle of the continuum are the situations defined as borderline states, which present identity and relationship problems.

Neutrality

Refers to the analyst's attitude that he or she should be neutral with respect to the patient's moral, religious, and social values, as well as with respect to the various contents of discourse, limiting his or her own bias.

Object

In psychoanalysis it is understood as an "object of affective investment", which can be a person or another living being, an idea or a concrete, emotionally important object for the subject. The object can be loved, hated, envied, and so on.

The concept of object that we will often use in the text, mind you, has nothing to do with treating others as objects, that is, with failing to recognise their dignity as human beings.

Oedipal triad
The Oedipus complex represents one of the cornerstones of Freudian psychoanalysis. It describes the 4- or 5-year-old child's love affair with one parent and fear of reprisal from the other parent. This triangle allows the child to develop the ability to think, tolerate frustrations, and psychically identify with one of the parents (usually one of the same biological sex).

Paranoia
A feeling or experience of persecution in which the person feels victimised.

Phantasmic experience
The way the patient experiences his or her unconscious fantasies.

Primary scene
The unconscious fantasy concerning the union of one's parents for one's own procreation.

Projection
The relatively primitive defence mechanism by which a desire, thought, or other mental content is considered as belonging to someone else rather than to ourselves.

Projective identification
A complex defence mechanism, quite primitive, by which one gets rid of a mental content by behaving towards another person in such a way as to prompt him or her to experience this feeling or thought.

Psychosomatics

The complex of theories and phenomena concerning the relationship between the body and mind, especially with regard to the influence of mind in the onset of physical disorders and diseases. Increasingly, today, mind and body are not seen as separate entities, but as different expressions of the individual, who reacts with complex psychosomatic responses to environmental stimulations.

Regression

Mechanism by which the psyche defends itself against frustration of its own desires by returning to an earlier, more reassuring, though more immature, state of development.

Removal

See **Repression**.

Representation

The ability of the psyche to visually or verbally depict an external object, affect, mood, or fantasy.

Repression

Fairly evolved defense mechanism by which the disturbing representation of a desire is censored and rendered unconscious.

Resistance

The conscious or unconscious obstacles to the development of the analytic process. Some theoretical models emphasise the resistances of the patient, others those experienced by the analytic couple.

Resonance

The analyst's listening that allows a share of the patient's experiences to be experienced emotionally to some extent.

Reverie

A state of receptivity of the mother or analyst to the unconscious communications of the child or patient. The use of reverie enables helping to process and transform raw sensory elements into experience.

Self

In psychoanalysis it has had several conceptual declinations. Generally, it is understood as the representation that the individual has of himself, or as the part of the psyche devoted to emotional experience. See also **grandiose self**.

Setting

The context within which the psychoanalytic process takes place. It consists mainly of the external elements, such as the room, the furniture, the schedule, the payments, and the analyst's internal setup towards working with the patient.

Splitting

Defence mechanism consisting of rigid compartmentalisation of the experience of self or object into good and bad, to protect the good parts from envy and destructiveness.

Stage (oral, anal, genital)

Psychosexual stages are defined as the different moments of infantile development, not to be considered rigidly or schematically, characterised by a prevailing mode of experiencing. In the oral stage this mode is incorporative, through sucking, biting, putting in the mouth, manipulating. In the anal (or urethral) stage there is play between holding and expelling. These are the pregenital stages, whilst in the genital stage there is the discovery of arousal of the genital areas.

Subject and person
See **Intersubjective and interpersonal**.

Superego
One of the three psychic instances identified by Freud along with ego and id. It oversees moral consciousness and limits ethically and socially unacceptable thoughts and behaviour. It is therefore responsible for moral, cultural, and social judgement and censorship activities.

Therapeutic alliance
The conscious collaborative relationship between patient and analyst is capable of motivating the therapeutic process, related suffering, and transference turmoil.

Topic
The representation of the psyche, according to Freud, in different systems as if they occupied a physical place. The first topic includes a conscious, preconscious, and unconscious participation; the second topic distinguishes the psychic instances of id, ego, and superego.

Transference
A key concept in psychoanalysis. The classic definition, now enriched and revised, is the repetition in adult life of infantile modes of relationship. Feelings, thoughts, and behaviours originally intended for parents or other primary figures are "transferred" to an object. The analyst can recognise the patient's transference and make therapeutic use of it (see also pp. 83–84 and 93–94 in Chapter 7).

Transpsychic
Type of psychic exchange whose bodily equivalents can be detected in the forced nurturing intrusions of mothers who impose the nipple in the infant's mouth with an excessive, imperious, and not at all empathetic adherence to their own private unconscious and/or indisputable behavioural assumptions, or to overly schematic nurturing protocols without attuning to the needs, desires, and conditions of the other (the child); or—even worse—in the penetrative violence of a *"penis-knife"* in rape. See also **Intrapsychic**.

References

Alexander, F. (1950). *Psychosomatic Medicine*. New York: W. W. Norton.

Bateman, A., & Fonagy, P. (2016). *Mentalization-Based Treatment for Personality Disorders: A Practical Guide*. Oxford: Oxford University Press.

Bolognini, S. (1994). Transference: Erotised, erotic, loving, affectionate. *International Journal of Psychoanalysis*, 75(1): 73–86.

Bolognini, S. (2005). Il bar nel deserto: simmetria e asimmetria nel trattamento di adolescenti difficili [The bar in the desert: Symmetry and asymmetry in the treatment of difficult adolescents]. *Rivista di Psicoanalisi*, 51(1): 33–44.

Bolognini, S. (2008). *Secret Passages: Theory and Technique of the Interpsychic Relationship*. London: Routledge.

Bolognini, S. (2012). The analyst's awkward gift: Balancing recognition of sexuality with parental protectiveness, *Psychoanalytic Quarterly*, LXXX(1): 33–54.

Bolognini, S. (2016). *Il sogno cento anni dopo [The Dream One Hundred Years Later]*. Milan: Mimesis.

Bolognini, S. (2019). *Vital Flows Between Self and Non-Self: The Interpsychic*. London: Routledge.

Busch, F. (2016). *Creating a Psychoanalytic Mind: A Method and a Psychoanalytic Theory*. Rome: Armando Editore.

Civitarese, G. (2016). *Truth and the Unconscious in Psychoanalysis*. London: Routledge.

Dement, W. C. (2001). *Il sonno e i suoi segreti [Sleep and its Secrets]*. Milan: Baldini & Castoldi.

Ferro, A., & Nicoli, L. (Ed.) (2017). *The New Analyst's Guide to the Galaxy.* London: Karnac.

Foresti, G. (2019). Arcana imperii: note su un disturbo collettivo nel funzionamento relazionale [Arcana imperii: Notes on a collective disorder in relational functioning]. *Psiche, 6*(2): 381–392.

Freud, S. (1905d). *Three Essays on the Theory of Sexuality. S. E., 7*: 123–246. London: Hogarth.

Gaddini, E. (1984). Se e come i nostri pazienti sono cambianti nei giorni presenti [If and how our patients are changing in the present day]. *Rivista di Psicoanalisi, 30*: 560–580.

Micati, L. (1993). Quanta realtà può essere tollerata? [How much reality can be tolerated?] *Rivista di Psicoanalisi, 39*: 153–163.

Ogden, T. H. (2013). Thomas H. Ogden in conversation with Luca Di Donna. *Rivista di Psicoanalisi, 59*: 625–641.

Ogden, T. H. (2019). Ontological psychoanalysis or "What do you want to be when you grow up?" *Psychoanalytic Quarterly, 88*: 661–684.

Peltz, R. (2015). What is "deep"? *Rivista di Psicoanalisi, 61*: 645–662.

Racamier, P. C. (1998). A psychotherapeutic treatment community: Reflections from a twenty-year experience. In: A. Ferruta, G. Foresti, E. Pedriali, & M. Vigorelli (Eds.), *The Therapeutic Community* (pp. 106–113). Milan: Raffaello Cortina Editore.

Spadoni, A. (1987). The obscure object of need. *Rivista di Psicoanalisi, 33*: 265–273.

Spazàl, S. (1990). Empathy and countertransference as constituent parts of psychoanalytic understanding. Proceedings of the Veneto-Emilia Psychoanalytic Meeting, 10 March 1990.

Steiner, J. (1993). *Psychic Retreats: Pathological Organizations in Psychotic, Neurotic and Borderline Patients.* New York: Taylor & Francis.

Wallerstein, R. S. (1988). One psychoanalysis or many? *International Journal of Psychoanalysis, 69*: 5–21.

Weintrobe, S. (Ed.) (2013). The difficult problem of anxiety when thinking about climate change. In: *Engaging With Climate Change: Psychoanalytic and Interdisciplinary Perspectives.* London: Routledge.

Index

Page numbers in **bold** indicate Glossary entries.